Praise for *The Power of Vital Force*

"The book you're holding in your hands right now contains an incredible distillation of what you might learn through years of studying many different Eastern traditions. But the single most precious thing you will get out of reading it is the knowledge that unconscious mental resistance and struggle makes everything you do harder than it needs to be."

— from the foreword by **Dave Asprey**,
founder and CEO of Bulletproof

"In this age of rampant burnout and stress, Patel shares a refreshing perspective on how we can use time-tested practices to seriously boost our energy, vitality, and well-being. Rich, practical, and life-changing wisdom!"

— **Emma Seppälä, Ph.D.**, author of *The Happiness Track*

"Human beings have labored immensely to explore the outer world; the continents, the oceans, the cosmos. Our creative enterprise and inquisitiveness has focused on the external—and we have failed to map the most mysterious terrain of all, the internal. . . . This book by Rajshree provides easy-to-use tools that actually optimize the internal landscape—our mental and emotional faculties. It provides the missing link to thriving both inside and out. It's the simple way to switch off your busy mind and turn on your power."

— **Jason Silva**, filmmaker, futurist, and former host of the Emmy-nominated *Brain Games*

"I had my team learn the tools to harness life energy and we found that with less effort we could achieve more. . . . High energy equals high impact. It naturally translates to greater self-empowerment, accountability, and generosity. One of the core statements at Panda is to 'Make Happy Happen.' The Power of Vital Force provides practical wisdom and techniques that naturally make happy happen."

— **Andrew Cherng**, founder and CEO of Panda Express

"A powerful guide full of actionable tools and practical timeless wisdom. If you are ready to think less and live more, read this book."

— **Bernardo Bonjean**, founder and CEO of Avante and entrepreneur

"If you are looking to change your life using meditation, don't settle for gimmicks and hype. Pick up this book and discover how ancient, time-tested tools of breath and meditation can bring vitality and clarity to your life."

— **Michael Edelstein**, former president of NBC Universal International Studios and executive producer of *Desperate Housewives*

"Neuroscience is finally catching up to what the wisdom of the East has been telling us for thousands of years. Vital force is the key to wellness. This book can up your game in every aspect of life."

— **Naveen Jain**, co-founder and CEO of Viome and author of *Moonshots: Creating a World of Abundance*

"The Power of Vital Force *is exceptional! . . . A true masterpiece that blends the 'art and science' of consciousness and what it takes to energize the human soul, to learn how to truly thrive in a way you could have never imagined."

— **Peter Cooper**, founder of Cooper Investors

"Finally, a book that gives the how-to's, not just what-to's. This book is filled with tools, practical insights, rooted in timeless wisdom that can enhance the physical and mental faculties with ease . . . and Rajshree with her deep wisdom and experience is the perfect exponent of these ancient truths."

— **Chandrika Tandon**, business leader, humanitarian, and Grammy-nominated artist

"A practical guidebook for anyone who would like to supercharge their life. The honest guidance is not only actionable, but refreshing and personable. I only wish I'd had a book like this when I started my career."

— **Rathi Murthy**, SVP and Chief Technology Officer of Gap, Inc.

"The Power of Vital Force *compiles all of Rajshree's wisdom and grace into easily applicable lessons. . . . Honestly, reading this book is the next best thing to working directly with Rajshree."

— **Jeremy Larner**, founder and president of JKL Worldwide and angel investor

The Power of

Vital Force

The Power of

Vital Force

ANCIENT SECRETS TO TRANSFORM HOW YOU THINK, FEEL, AND ACT

Rajshree Patel

HAY HOUSE, INC.
Carlsbad, California • New York City
London • Sydney • New Delhi

Copyright © 2019 by Rajshree Patel

Published in the United States by: Hay House, Inc.: www.hayhouse.com®
Published in Australia by: Hay House Australia Pty. Ltd.: www.hayhouse.com.au
Published in the United Kingdom by: Hay House UK, Ltd.: www.hayhouse.co.uk
Published in India by: Hay House Publishers India: www.hayhouse.co.in

Cover design: The Book Designers • *Interior design:* Nick C. Welch
Indexer: Carol Roberts

All rights reserved. No part of this book may be reproduced by any me-chanical, photographic, or electronic process, or in the form of a phonographic recording; nor may it be stored in a retrieval system, transmitted, or otherwise copied for public or private use—other than for "fair use" as brief quotations embodied in articles and reviews—without prior written permission of the pub-lisher.

The author of this book does not dispense medical advice or prescribe the use of any technique as a form of treatment for physical, emotional, or medical problems without the advice of a physician, either directly or indirectly. The in-tent of the author is only to offer information of a general nature to help you in your quest for emotional, physical, and spiritual well-being. In the event you use any of the information in this book for yourself, the author and the publisher assume no responsibility for your actions.

**Cataloging-in-Publication Data is on file
at the Library of Congress**

Tradepaper ISBN: 978-1-4019-5634-9
E-book ISBN: 978-1-4019-5633-2
Audiobook ISBN: 978-1-4019-5632-5

10 9 8 7 6 5 4 3 2 1
1st edition, August 2019
2nd edition, April 2021

Printed in the United States of America

To the innate resilience of life itself

Contents

Foreword   xi
Introduction: My Story and Your Journey   xv

PART I: TURN ON YOUR POWER

Chapter 1:   Energy Is Life   3
Chapter 2:   Beyond Belief   21
Chapter 3:   Ancient Biohacking   41

PART II: BRAIN DRAIN

Chapter 4:   A Machine Called Mind   53
Chapter 5:   The Past Is Present   75
Chapter 6:   The Mindfulness Trap   97

PART III: REBOOT AND RECHARGE

Chapter 7:   The Secret of Life   117
Chapter 8:   Meditation for Busy People   137
Chapter 9:   Living Your Inner Superpowers   153

PART IV: UPGRADE YOUR OPERATING SYSTEM

Chapter 10:   Mastering Your Mind-Set   181
Chapter 11:   From Fighting to Flowing   187
Chapter 12:   Cutting Craving   207

PART V: THE BIG MIND

Chapter 13:   Undivided Mind   221
Chapter 14:   It's All Connected   237

Last Word   255

More for You to Explore   259
Endnotes   261
Index   263
Acknowledgments   273
About the Author   275

Foreword

For the past two decades, I've worked to become a higher-performing, better human being by any means possible. At first, that meant doing the things that are supposed to work in a place like Silicon Valley. Working harder. Studying. Pushing. Staying up late. Getting an Ivy League MBA. Making millions before I turned 27. Unfortunately, I was exhausted and miserable, not to mention angry, without even realizing it most of the time.

I went on to spend more than $1 million improving my biology at every level, from the sub-cellular all the way to the highest spiritual levels I could find. Along the way, I created the modern field of biohacking: the art and science of changing the environment inside and outside of our bodies so that we have full control of our own biology.

It even led me to create Bulletproof, my company dedicated to human performance (and butter in coffee) that has served about 200 million cups of brain-enhancing coffee. I've written best-selling science books about the brain, interviewed hundreds of researchers on consciousness and biology on Bulletproof Radio, my Webby award–winning podcast, and started a neuroscience facility for upgrading the human brain.

The deeper essence of the things that powered that learning and achievement—and the connective tissue behind all forms of biohacking and personal growth—are here for you in this book.

At the start of my path, I began by pushing the limits of what I'd learned as a computer hacker. I went to doctors and psychologists and exhausted the things that were supposed to work to give me energy and health. I ended up more successful but still angry for no apparent reason, still tired, and no happier. One day, an engineer from India I worked with at a startup told me about a new kind of meditation he thought I'd like. Figuring it was worth a try, I showed up. There were flowers and candles and I arrived with a skeptical computer hacker mind. Even though there was something valuable dangling right in front of my face during the course, I rejected it because I judged it through my preconceived Western notions.

And then I rediscovered it two years later, when the CEO of the startup said, "Dave, come to this meditation training for executives at the home of one of the top executives from Intel." Who turns down an invitation like that from the boss? I spent a weekend learning what tools from the Vedic tradition, specifically The Art of Living Happiness Program, could do for me. As a result of that weekend, I added those exercises to my "stack" of high-performance behaviors and practiced them daily for more than five years.

At 7 A.M. every Saturday morning, I'd meet a dozen other executives to do the Vedic breathing and meditation exercises. My friend Prabakar, a well-known CTO, put it best when he said, "I can't explain why breathing in a group like this works, but it's like taking a mental shower for the week. I'm nicer at work."

Those breathing and meditation exercises were my introduction to the vast science of energy management recorded in the ancient teachings of the Vedic tradition. As you'll learn in this book, the wisdom of Vedanta goes far beyond daily practices for performance and stress relief. The powerful meditation and breathwork techniques that I learned barely scratch the surface of what's in the book. Included within this book, you will find a comprehensive system for physical and mental enhancement and human thriving.

You might even think of the Vedic tradition, as the book says, as "ancient biohacking." While our technology and understanding of our own biology have advanced by quantum leaps since the time of the Vedas, these thousands-of-years-old principles and techniques are still unparalleled in terms of the wisdom and tools they offer for upgrading the mind, body and spirit.

The book you're holding in your hands right now contains an incredible distillation of what you might learn through years of studying many different Eastern traditions. But the single most precious thing you will get out of reading it is the knowledge that unconscious mental resistance and struggle makes everything you do harder than it needs to be. With great wisdom and a sense of humor, Rajshree Patel will help you to understand how your "machine called mind" is creating problems in your life—and how to turn off your busy mind to turn on your true power.

What I've found through years of biohacking, and what this book describes with great clarity, is that mind and energy are two sides of the same coin. When you're effectively managing your own mind, your energy levels skyrocket. And when you're keeping your energy levels high, your mental performance—including thoughts, emotions, awareness, and outlook—naturally increases. Your mind-set shifts from one of resistance and struggle to one of acceptance, gratitude, and strength. This virtuous cycle is one of the greatest secrets to high performance, and in this book, you'll learn how to master this two-pronged approach to excelling and thriving.

Who you are is a being of infinite power and potential. Unlocking that potential isn't about self-improvement or self-help. Instead, as Patel writes, it's about *self-awareness*. It's about upgrading from the "small mind" of conditioned thinking, emotions tied to the past and future, and limiting mind-sets to what Vedanta calls the "Big Mind" of unlimited intelligence, love, and potentiality.

By contemplating and applying the precious knowledge in these pages, you will learn to make everything in your life easier than you think is possible. Relationships. Jobs. Family. Creativity. Happiness. And maybe even doing something more game-changing than you've ever thought possible. It doesn't come from hard work or more effort. It comes from embracing the power that is your birthright: the energy of life itself, the power that gave you life and that keeps you alive. That energy is *vital force*.

I invite you to step into these pages with an open mind so that you can learn how good it feels when things in your life happen with ease and excitement.

Dave Asprey

Founder and CEO of Bulletproof
and *New York Times* best-selling author

Introduction

My Story and Your Journey

The great passion driving my life has been the mystery of a single question: *Who am I?*

Even as a child, I wondered what it is that makes people go through the same circumstances in completely different ways. I suppose I came to this inquiry by growing up observing the harsh realities of life in rural India, seeing many who regularly went to bed hungry—myself included—later go on to thrive in their lives, while others who seemingly had it all lived in a state of constant struggle. I asked myself: *What is it about ourselves that seems to determine the quality of our lives?*

I have spent the last 30 years of my life traveling around the globe working in the field of human potential as a teacher, speaker, and coach. I've been exploring, at an experiential and practical level, the mystery of the Self, both in my personal life and with others. This simple question—*Who am I?*—has transformed not only my own daily life, career, and relationships but also the lives of hundreds of thousands of people around the globe, from Fortune 500 CEOs to homemakers to students to actors and artists to war veterans. I have watched one individual after another effortlessly harness their deeper potential, power, and presence to thrive in their lives on a physical, mental, emotional, and spiritual level as they discover who they really are. That's why I wrote this book: to share with you the wisdom and tools that have proved invaluable to me and countless others along this journey of Self.

One of the first things that I discovered along this journey is that we have all been fed a great lie. Our parents, teachers, and society, knowingly or perhaps unknowingly, have fed us the biggest bunch of B.S. you can imagine. That great lie is this: We have to effort, we have to work hard and think hard, in order to do or have anything great in our lives.

What I've learned over all these years is that being truly happy, connected, dynamic, and thriving has very little to do with thinking or hard work. Look around, really look! Most people who achieve true success in life (and I'm talking about *life*, not just work) aren't killing themselves toiling day and night, nor are they wasting their time strategizing their way to the top. What they've created and how they live is not only, or even primarily, the product of hard work. It's something else—something much bigger than effort on a physical or mental level.

What is that something? It's a certain magic quality, an indescribable magnetism, that we feel in the presence of those who are truly successful inside and out; those who are vibrant, alive, and dynamic. We might describe it as mojo, chutzpah, or just plain energy. It's the ability to go for it—whatever "it" might be—without hesitation or doubt, with full clarity and a *yes* mind. This is not something that comes from outside. It's something that we, *you*, were born with. As children, we all had this inner presence, power, and *aliveness*. You don't need to achieve it, you just have to reclaim it.

The secret to thriving is not hard work or strategic thinking. It's the effortless power of life itself—the life that you were born with. It is the innate energy and intelligence that surrounds and interpenetrates every particle of our existence. It is who and what we are. We simply have to know it, claim it, and it will work for us and with us.

The intention of this book is to empower you in your journey to reclaiming that power. My wish and intention is that it will offer you valuable guidance and support along your path of self-discovery, as you move ever closer to the perfection that lies within you.

~

When I was younger, I first started asking this question of who am I on the level of my cultural identity. Born in Uganda and raised between rural India and New York City, I was a first-generation American immigrant. *Who am I, Indian or American?* It progressed to asking who am I as a woman: *Who am I as a daughter, a sister, a potential wife?* After I graduated from law school, I would ask myself, *Who am I as a lawyer? Am I a prosecutor or a defense attorney?* The question moved inward from there: *Am I just my body? Am I my thoughts? Or am I something beyond that?*

In my younger years, it felt like a burden to ask this question of who I am because I felt caught between two cultural identities. I didn't really fit into either. On the one hand, I was raised in America, to choose a life partner whenever you wanted (and that's if you even wanted one); on the other hand, my Indian background said that getting married and having kids was the only possible life path. Saying no to marriage and kids wasn't much of an option.

As the only living daughter in my family, I felt a lot of pressure and expectation from my parents about who I had to be, and let me tell you, I was anything *but* the model Indian girl. I was always independent and rebellious, with a sharp tongue and a temper. When I was seven years old, my aunt got married in a village in Gujarat, where I grew up. In those days there was a practice of the bride's family having to offer a dowry to the groom's family. Each time the couple circled around the fire in the process of taking their vows, the bride's family would offer something of value—perhaps a watch, or a gold chain, or a silver bracelet. I was sitting by myself on the top of the roof watching the whole spectacle. Suddenly, in the middle of the ceremony, the groom's mother said, "We don't want *that*, we want *this*, or else this wedding will not happen." My grandmother couldn't afford what was being demanded, which obviously put the family in a tight spot. When I saw what was happening, I shouted down from the rooftop, "We don't want to sell our aunt! Take your son and go away. You should be giving *us* money!" My uncle came running over and dragged me away.

Most parents have some expectations for their children, and Indian parents tend to have a *lot* of expectations. You probably won't be surprised to hear that I fought against my parents' expectations for years. My parents wanted me to get married before I went to university or did anything else with my life. They were afraid I would become "too independent" and break tradition. Instead, I went to law school, without their approval, and took out student loans to pay my way through. In my early twenties, at their behest, I actually went to India to consider an arranged marriage, and I gave up after six days of asking myself what the hell I was doing there! Those six days set the direction of my life. I decided to go against their wishes, fight the cultural battles. I stayed single, completed grad school, and ultimately moved across the country to work as a federal prosecutor in California and later as a prosecutor with the Los Angeles District Attorney's office. A few years later, my life took an even more dramatic and unexpected shift when I left behind criminal law for what you might call "natural law"—the study of our inner world of mind, emotion, and spirit.

It has not been easy to let go of the hardwiring that told me who I was supposed to be, the conditioning that led me to put myself into boxes like "Indian," "daughter," "high achiever," "immigrant," and "lawyer." My childhood, my gender, my ethnicity, my traumas, and my accomplishments—like yours— have all shaped an identity and belief system that have served me well to achieve and succeed by conventional standards. But these identifications also became the limits and boundaries of my own potential. It has not been easy to "lay down," as the sages and mystics say, and to step out of the comfort zone that I once knew as myself. But I now know that for anything truly great to happen in our lives, we must rediscover who we really are. We must rewire our identities to be more than the sum total of our experiences that have come and gone. We have to rewrite the programs of our minds that have been conditioned to think, feel, perceive, and believe a certain way.

I'm neither a scientist nor a mystic, but after 30 years of empirical observation and study, I do know this much: there is more to life, more to us, than just what we see, hear, touch, and feel.

I have never been one to accept anything at face value. As a lawyer, evidence is everything to me. The only language of spirituality that ever worked for me was my own experience. Throughout my own journey, I have had to experience for myself who I am in a larger sense, beyond my cultural identity, beyond the roles I've played in my life, beyond matter, beyond thoughts, and ultimately beyond my own mind. Along the way I have discovered a power and potential that serves to uplift and support not only my life but the lives of tens of thousands of other people I've been fortunate enough to work with. Today, *Who am I?* is not just a question for me, it's a wonder.

The pragmatist in me has been curious about what science as much as mysticism has to say about this question of who we are. Of course, I'm neither a scientist nor a mystic, but after 30 years of empirical observation and study, I do know this much: there is more to life, more to us, than just what we see, hear, touch, and feel. I know that we are both matter and energy. We are both body and mind. We are both intellect and emotion. We are both seen and unseen. We are both solid and space. We seek both success and significance through meaning in life.

The problem is that we have been conditioned to experience life in a purely material way. We barely stop to recognize feelings and emotions, let alone the field of energy and consciousness underlying all of life that scientists and sages around the world have spoken of for thousands of years. We have not been trained to turn within. It wasn't always this way: traditionally in India, young people were educated for 12 years in the material sciences—math, science, reading, and language—and simultaneously for 12 years in the inner sciences of spirit, heart, mind, energy, and consciousness. This second school was called *gurukula*, the schooling of mind. Study of nature, mind, and spirit was prevalent in many ancient civilizations. In India it was present from ancient times up until the colonial period. But that tradition has long been lost. In our modern lives, we are taught to pay attention only to the surface level of reality, and as a result, we've shifted our center of identity to what we can see, hear, touch, and feel. We are absorbed in the world of matter, with eyes open and our attention turned outward most of the time. With eyes closed, we are asleep to the deeper, unseen reality of life that lies beneath the surface. But we have to look inside to tune in to the frequency of who we are, to recognize our greater potential and the field of possibilities that underlies our external material reality.

Usually we turn within only in moments of crisis or hardship, or because of a stroke of luck. In my case it was both.

My stroke of luck came on a spring evening in Los Angeles in 1989, when I was in my mid-twenties. I was on my way to what I thought was a music concert. You can imagine my surprise when I arrived at the "concert" to discover not the Indian sitarist Ravi Shankar but instead the spiritual master Sri Sri Ravi Shankar. At that point in my life, I had no interest in gurus or spirituality, but by the time I caught on to my mistake, it was too late to leave without making a scene. So I sat there rolling my eyes and making silent judgments about what the master was saying for most of the talk. His comments about life, success, happiness, and the nature of reality were nice ideas, perhaps, but to me they felt cheesy and idealistic, somehow disconnected from real life down here on planet Earth. I'll tell you the whole story of that fateful first encounter a little later on, but for now, just know that I decided in spite of my "better judgment" to join a workshop that Sri Sri was leading the following weekend.

In the workshop, I started learning the philosophy and tools of the Vedic tradition of India, in particular a breathwork practice that had been passed down since ancient times. On the second day, something happened that I suppose you could describe as a metaphysical experience—something that I still to this day don't have language for. Although words fall far short, what I can tell you is that I had an experience of *who I am* beyond every possible identification, boundary, and limitation. For the span of perhaps a few moments, I experienced an explosion of unlimited energy, unlimited awareness, and a sense of love and gratitude so immense that it could not be contained—a love without a particular object, a love that knew no bounds. I was weeping internally but without sorrow.

Or at least I thought it was internally. I didn't realize in that moment that I had been crying out loud during breathing meditation. I thought it was all in my head! It felt like I was dreaming, but with eyes open. It was that vivid. When I finally opened my eyes, I noticed that everyone was sitting up; they had shared their experiences with one another, and now they were all staring at me, my face flooded with tears. As I looked around the room, I honestly didn't know if I was outside my eyes, looking in, or if I was inside my body, looking out of my eyes. Imagine being in a room where the entire wall is a window, so you almost don't know if you're inside or outside anymore— that's what this was like. I had just had the clearest experience that *who I am* is energy that is full of love and awareness beyond belief. I felt that I could be in any place at any moment. I understood for the first time that there is something that travels faster than light—my mind. It's me! It's *us*. Our minds, our awareness, can be anywhere at any time; we just don't see it because we're focused on the body. In this moment, I knew without a doubt: I am not just my body. I am something much more powerful and indescribable that is housed in and around this body.

I had no way of explaining this to myself. The result of the experience—*that* I could explain. It was a very clear sense of an almost superhuman self-empowerment. Once I saw this deeper power and potential within myself, all my limiting beliefs dropped. Just like that, they were gone. Without even being consciously aware of what was happening, I stopped saying *I can't, I won't, I don't do that, I don't know if it's possible.* I was suddenly redefining myself—and not based on another belief system. I suddenly saw myself beyond anything I could ever imagine or anything I have ever seen in another person. I have admired a lot of people who are role models and visionary leaders, from dear friends who survived years in Auschwitz, to my father who had the spirit of a lion and overcame the most adverse situations in his life, to people like Gandhi, Nelson Mandela, and Martin Luther King, Jr., who lived with a resounding spirit that said anything is possible. That weekend, I had the sense that whatever they have, I have in me. I suddenly had confidence, clarity, and a sense of myself that was beyond anything I could have imagined.

Now, bear in mind that my lawyerly brain still wasn't interested in anything metaphysical. As powerful as the experience was, part of me blew it off as some strange fluke. But what *was* interesting to me was what happened at work the next day and over the course of the next few weeks. From that Monday onward, my efficiency was through the roof. Case files that had previously taken me four hours to analyze, process, and put together I could now complete in an hour. I'd finish 25 files by myself in the same amount of time it took my colleagues to complete maybe 10 or 11. The mental chatter, the noise in my mind that was so normal to me, all but disappeared. I was so in the zone that I would put together the file without even knowing what I was doing.

Even so, begrudgingly, I took another step and signed up for a 10-day silent retreat at the insistence of the friend I'd brought to the course. I didn't go on the retreat thinking it was about spirituality. My main motivation was my newfound productivity and imagining how much more efficient I might become if I did the work for a full 10 days. Yet, while I went into the course with that goal, in the background I was trying to figure out what I wanted. I was scared to death about the notion of marriage based on what I'd seen of traditional marriages in India with fixed roles of husband and wife, along with the divorce rate I'd witnessed in America. My dad was still calling me at the office every week with a new marriage prospect, but I kept resisting. *Do I want to focus on my career and not have kids at all?* I didn't have any good answers to these questions.

I remember going to a popular bookstore in L.A. called The Bodhi Tree and seeing a wall of saints and sages. I wondered to myself, *If one of these people existed in my lifetime, would I see life differently?* But I was certain that those stories of yogic masters were just fictional stories of imaginary times past, like Noah's ark or the loaves and fishes. I never really thought that it was possible for one to be self-actualized on this planet.

This gives you a sense of my state of mind when I embarked on that silence retreat and suddenly had one of the rudest awakenings of my life. Primed by my experience at the first workshop, by the end of three or four days I had discovered a whole new world that was far bigger than anything I could see or possibly understand. I experienced a wake-up call that rang through my head like a loudspeaker: *Reality—the world I see, touch, feel, and experience in front of me—is nothing more than my internal perception of it.* I saw that each one of us is walking around inside of our own reality. In some sense, this made reality not a reality at all. What I heard in the silence was that whatever was happening around me—no matter how fixed and determinate it seemed—was a reflection of what was happening inside my own mind. It was my mind, more than anything else, that determined how and what I experienced in my life.

It was at that moment I began my journey inward, but it was not without conflict. That journey has meant fighting tooth and nail to break free from my mind's conditioning and limiting belief systems. The sages say that you have to "lay yourself down" to discover, to do, and to be great. Well, let me tell you, it has been *hell* to lay myself down because I have such a strong left brain. My rational, skeptical, lawyerly mind fought me every single step of this spiritual journey as I've been pushed to expand from the I-achievement-oriented, I-results-focused, pragmatic Indian girl that my parents taught me to be. I was trained very, very well by my parents to achieve in the external world. That training has served me well and continues to serve me. But what has accelerated my success, deep joy, and sense of significance in my life much further is adopting a new set of tools, outlook, and wisdom to help me navigate my inner world.

Defying my parents once again, I suddenly left my career in law—and I mean *suddenly*. After the silence course, when Sri Sri invited me to join him in India, I made plans to spend six weeks there as a kind of "break" before I entered my thirties and got saddled with all the responsibilities of adult life. Well, six weeks turned into five years studying and teaching meditation, breathwork, and Vedic philosophy in India. My parents thought I had gone mad. *You did WHAT?! You walked away from your profession? That's insane!* And I went to India, of all places! They'd left India to be in America, and here I was, going back to some podunk village to sit in silence and do nothing all day. That's what it looked like to them.

Over the course of the years that followed, I went on to launch and grow Sri Sri's organization The Art of Living, a foundation dedicated to sharing the wisdom and techniques of the Vedic tradition to help people live happier, more successful, and more peaceful lives. I established an infrastructure that led to opening, in rapid succession, one Art of Living center after another throughout the world, leading to significant growth. From India I would go to Hong Kong, Japan, South America, Europe, the U.S., and Canada, establishing more and more new centers, studying the Vedic tradition and setting up events. As soon as one center was set up, I'd move on to the next city or country, the next new center. The years flew by as I traveled across more than 35 countries spreading Vedic teachings, opening hundreds of meditation centers, and impacting thousands of people's lives, all the while with that little voice of my parents in the back of my head saying, *Who the hell does that, following some unknown guru and setting up centers for him all over the world? And as a single woman?*

There was a greater power that was propelling all of this, and I was connected to it. My energy was pulsating and vibrating at a frequency I'd never experienced before. My radio was tuned in. I would meet the right person, and the thing that needed to happen would happen. With no events coordinator, no marketing, and no resources, I was organizing and teaching three courses a day, with over 300 people showing up for each course.

Within a few short years, a "start-up" organization called The Art of Living expanded from India to a global operation serving hundreds of thousands of people of all ages and all walks of life. I went on to become the trainer of trainers, as well as to develop and lead more targeted programs on corporate culture, leadership, conscious parenting, relationships, and other advanced courses designed to expand human potential and power. Today, the little start-up I once knew has grown to more than 150 countries, with tens of thousands of teachers around the world.

It's difficult for me to even quantify how all of this happened. Art of Living started with an unknown guru and four teachers. I was fortunate to be one of the four. Now, we have 50,000 teachers in India alone. Today, Sri Sri, who was known to only pockets of people in his home country, is internationally beloved and celebrated by millions—not only as a yogic master but also as a humanitarian. He's become an ambassador of peace throughout the world, working with heads of state and even aiding in peace negotiations in countries like Sri Lanka, Pakistan, and Colombia.

For this to happen, I had to continually move myself beyond the limits of my own thinking. At the beginning, it could never have occurred to me that Art of Living would become a massive, global operation that would make an impact not only on people's internal lives but also outwardly through social impact programs in such areas as prisoner rehabilitation (IAHV Prison Program), inner-city youth empowerment (YES! for Schools), post-traumatic stress relief for war veterans (Project Welcome Home Troops), disaster and trauma relief, and grassroots efforts providing food, clothing, clean water, and electricity. The list goes on: planting over a million trees to combat climate change, supporting women's empowerment, and much more. The organization today is a far cry from my little idea of a guru and his disciples sitting in a straw hut in the mountains somewhere. It's an organization that has had a tremendous social impact on all levels, one that defines spirituality and its mission by seeking to create a stress-free, violence-free world.

"Vital force," or "life energy," is the fundamental energy within and around us that gives us life and sustains our lives. When we're tapped into that source, we bring more energy—more life— to everything we touch.

But again, it wasn't just *me* that was making all of this happen. I was connected to the energy of life itself, and it was guiding me at every step to create a life beyond anything I had ever imagined for myself. That may sound a little woo-woo, perhaps even a little cheesy, but I've never stopped being a pragmatic person. Even today, I translate the connection I'm describing into a way of being more alive, vibrant, and productive. This force of life that I was tuned in to in Sri Sri's workshop was the same thing that was helping me process my case files faster. It was the same energy that was making me happier, more vibrant, more enthusiastic and energized in my daily life. It was reducing my stress levels and making me more mindful and aware. Everything I wanted was coming from the same source. This force that I'm talking about is what the Vedic tradition calls "vital force," or "life energy." It's the fundamental energy within and around us that gives us life and sustains our lives. When we're tapped into that source, we bring more energy—more *life*—to everything we touch. It's an extremely powerful force that's behind all our physical and mental functions.

Your Journey through the Book

My big wake-up call back in 1989 taught me that while we look for answers outside of ourselves, both the cause and the solution of what we're experiencing lie within. We constantly seek to regulate our inner landscape of thoughts, emotions, mind, and perception by managing the things and people around us. We look for reasons, cause and effect in things, situations, and people outside. Looking through our own eyes, through the lens of our own conditioning, we never consider that perhaps *we* are creating the results that appear in the world around us. We never stop to ask whether the limitations we experience are coming from within rather than from without.

When we do acknowledge this possibility, it forces us to take responsibility for the way we are creating our reality at all times. It can be a painful truth to face, but with it comes a great secret: We can influence the nature of our reality and results by changing the way we look out of our own eyes. We can change the conditioned "I" that has its existence based on other people's passed-on notions of reality, truth, right and wrong, should be and should not be. We can break through the limits of our own beliefs and thought patterns to take in this greater force of life that wants nothing more than to support and uplift us.

This book is filled with simple, effortless tools designed to melt the conditioned "I," what I call "the iceberg of the mind," so that you can tap into the greater force of life within you. It's a practical pathway to the unlimited source of energy and intelligence that exists beyond the thinking and reasoning mind. It is a way to get out of your own way, to "lay down," so that great things can happen in your life—so that you can tap into the energy of life within yourself to re-create your life, your reality, your Self.

What do I mean by Self with a capital *S*? I'm talking about the part of you that is unlimited, that is pure potentiality. The Vedic tradition says this Self has three qualities: unlimited energy, unlimited intelligence or knowingness, and the unlimited potentiality of what we can call "love," "connectivity," or "belongingness." It describes these three qualities by the word *satchitananda*, "existence, consciousness, bliss." It's the experience that I had of existing beyond my body, my thoughts, my emotions, my own catalogue of memories and life experiences. What I tapped into during that experience was this Self with a capital *S*: the sub-subatomic aspect of who I am, below even the quantum level of my own identity.

As powerful as the experience was, my rational mind couldn't help but dismiss it as some kind of strange momentary fluke. But when I started to see this same experience of Self happen to thousands of people, I could no longer deny its power. I saw it happen to people of every walk of life in America, in Germany, in India, in South America, and all over the world. It's undeniable that we are far more than what we measure—but to realize and experience our unlimited nature, we have to explore the ways that we have become limited by our own thinking.

To access the deeper potentiality that is at your core—and to create any kind of real change in your life—it's not enough to just think about it on the surface of your mind, as a concept in your intellect. First you have to erase the mind's old, backed-up hard drive. You have to make some space in the memory. You need to create a tiny crack in the iceberg where the ocean can flow through. If you take a dip in the ocean of consciousness that surrounds the iceberg, it will go 10 times as far in supporting you to float. The tools in this book are designed to create not just cracks in the iceberg but a rift the size of the Grand Canyon. Read the book, and then, if you wish, visit RajshreePatel.com to learn about an online course that will guide you to integrate this wisdom into your daily life. Even if you use just one or two of the tools, you will already be transforming how you think, feel, and act. You will find a way to control your inner landscape of thoughts, emotions, and sensations. You will experience what it means to have less stress, more efficiency, and more ease. You will live in the moment by letting go of what is dead and gone. You will enhance your performance by becoming more mindful and connected to yourself and those around you. As you learn to better manage your own mind, you will conserve and enhance your energy, and as your energy rises, your mind will be naturally and effortlessly uplifted. It's a virtuous cycle that we'll explore in depth in this book.

What we're talking about here isn't self-help or self-improvement. It's more a process of self-realizing. We're not trying to make ourselves better, because we are already perfect. We're just reconnecting to who we really are by peeling back the layers of conditioning that cloud the perfection that exists at our core. The first step to living from our core essence, our innate *consciousness*, is to become aware of what's clouding it and getting in the way.

We're not trying to make ourselves better, because we are already perfect. We're just reconnecting to who we really are by peeling back the layers of conditioning that cloud the perfection that exists at our core.

We begin in Part I, "Turn On Your Power," by reacquainting ourselves with this thing called "vital force," the energy of life within and around us. You'll learn about how this energy is different from what you've been taught to think of as energy, and you'll discover why it's so important to recharge your own internal batteries. In Part II, "Brain Drain," we'll look at the biggest energy hog of our entire system—the machine called "mind"—and we'll closely examine how the workings of our mental machinery are draining our batteries and reducing our potentiality.

In Part III, "Reboot and Recharge," you will learn how to get your mojo back using a set of simple and effective ancient tools for conserving and recharging the battery of your innate life force. These techniques have been passed down for thousands of years to help us tap into the *source* of energy itself in order to uplift us on every level: physically, mentally, emotionally, creatively, and spiritually. What we're talking about in the broader sense is not just enhancing our energy and becoming more effective in all we do, but embracing our true power as co-creators, working with the energy of life itself to manifest our desires on a material level. When we align ourselves with the flow of life, we can start to organize and reorganize the particles of matter around us based on our own intentions. The embodied practices of the *yama* and *niyama* described in Chapter 9 will create the driving force behind the intentions that we seek to manifest. These embodied practices help us to open our hearts and operate from a place of uplifted emotion and attention, strengthening our intention and giving us the force to reconfigure our reality.

Armed with these tools, we're ready to go even deeper. In Part IV, "Upgrade Your Operating System," we'll explore the two core mind-sets that we spend most of our lives operating from and that are responsible for all of our unhappiness. We'll learn to shift and transform these mind-sets through the power of our awareness, to return the mind to its most expansive and uplifted state: a beginner's mind that is totally in the flow of the present moment. In Part V, "The Big Mind," we'll arrive at our core: consciousness, or what Vedanta calls *satchitananda*. In the Vedic tradition, energy and consciousness are two sides of a coin. By enhancing our innate energy, we are also expanding our consciousness. And as our consciousness expands, we find what we're really seeking in life: to feel connected to the whole, to be a part of something greater.

I'm grateful to you for joining me in this journey of Self that's been my mission for the past 30 years. To succeed, all you need is an open mind and an open heart. Expect the unexpected. Deep self-reflection is a critical element of this process, so please take your time and allow yourself the space to digest these ideas and see how they apply to your life. Be willing to completely change the way you see yourself as your awareness begins to transform, and, of course, remember that everything you need is already there inside of you. You're not fixing any part of yourself or introducing anything that's not already there. You're simply reconnecting to the unlimited power and potential that is your human birthright.

PART I

TURN ON YOUR POWER

CHAPTER 1

Energy Is Life

Long before I began my study of the inner world, a rather extreme moment in my early legal career became a pivotal point in my journey of Self. When I was around 24 years old, I went on a field trip to a coroner's office as a way to better prepare myself to handle murder trials. I had never been to one before and arrived there without any expectations. As I was led down the stairs, I noticed lots of what I presumed were covered bodies on either side of me. I didn't think much of it. Then, I arrived in a room, in the center of which was a table supporting the body of a woman who appeared to be eight or nine months pregnant. The coroner began an autopsy with a traditional Y incision. As he continued cutting, examining and measuring each organ, I was perplexed. To me, this woman looked as if she were sleeping.

At one point, the coroner removed the woman's uterus and cut it open to remove the body of a baby boy. He pulled him out by one of the legs and placed him on a scale, saying out loud, "Seven-point-three pounds." Now my brain was really short-circuiting. *Why is he grabbing the baby like that? What is going on with this woman?*

The cause of death was a ricocheted bullet that hit her heart and then traveled to the baby's heart. Part of me knew she was dead, as was the baby, but the death wasn't computing in my brain. She looked just like any other pregnant woman. I felt somehow disconnected from the reality that she was not alive. At this point my mind began rolling into a stream of questions around the difference between life and death—not in some esoteric way, but on a practical level, about what it really means to be alive, to *have life*. All of this woman's organs and the baby's organs were healthy, but she was not living. She just looked to me as if she were sleeping, but clearly any level of movement, consciousness, or vitality was absent. I couldn't help but ask myself, *What is it that makes us alive? What is the difference between being alive and just existing?*

And I couldn't help but begin to ask the same question about myself. *What am I doing with my life? Am I walking around fully alive, or am I somehow asleep?* I thought about how the woman had lived her life before it was gone. I wondered, *Did she really live her life, or did she just go through the motions of it? To what degree was she really alive while she had her life? How alive am I as I walk through my own life?*

Before we go on, I would like you to ask yourself the same question I asked myself: *At this moment, how alive do I feel?* Do you spring out of bed full of life and excitement to see your partner next to you, challenged by the day ahead and grateful to be on this planet orbiting in space, or do you drag yourself out of bed already stressed about the day ahead? The way you answer these questions is a direct measure of the quality of not only your external life but the life within you.

Fuel for Life

The experience at the coroner's office rather unexpectedly triggered a deep line of inquiry about what it really meant for me to be alive. I had it "all" in my life, but somehow I felt there was something lacking. It didn't occur to me at the time, but the quality of our inner life, what's going on in our minds, is directly related to the level of energy that we have. I hadn't realized it, that this energy that keeps us alive and vibrant—what the ancient traditions call "life energy," or vital force—is a fundamental force that we can all easily tap into. It's a simple equation: the more energy you have, the more *alive* you are. Energy is life, and life is energy! The more energy you have, the more positive and expansive your state of mind is and the more you thrive.

I'll fill you in on a big secret: *everything is energy*. We know this from modern physics, and long before that, we knew it from the wisdom of the ancients. Human beings—and all living things, in fact—are made up of physical units of electromagnetic energy. Your cell membranes are designed to conduct electricity. Your heart and brain are electrical systems, and doctors can measure their wave activity using EKG and EEG machines. On the most macro scale, it's electromagnetic energy that determines the movements of the stars and planets. On the most microscopic scale, the tiniest particles, atoms, are made up of protons and electrons that have a positive or negative energetic charge.

If you stop for a moment to think about it, you'll see that energy provides the fuel for everything in life, from plants and animals to iPhones to light bulbs to the human body. It's obvious that everything we do requires energy, from blinking our eyes to walking, talking, thinking, digesting food, or having a creative breakthrough. We require energy to function on every level of our being: physical, mental, emotional, spiritual, and sexual. The more optimally you want each level to function, the more vital fuel is required. But for the most part, we've never stopped to look at the connection between this energy of life and the quality of our lives. It may sound obvious, but no one has ever taught us, not at home or in school, how to maximize our performance and quality of life by harnessing it.

Energy is the fuel that runs not only our bodies but also our minds and emotions. We vibrate with it. We project it into our words, actions, thoughts, looks, and feelings. This energy of life, this vital force, is *aliveness* itself. To the degree you are tapped into it and accessing it, to that degree you thrive— *thrive* meaning you are growing, flourishing, blossoming, and evolving. To the degree that you are depleted of it, to that degree you struggle, become weakened and ineffective, and get stuck.

Let's face it: when you're tired and depleted, when you don't have the energy to get out of bed or you feel overwhelmed by the demands of your day, it really doesn't matter what's going on in your life—the glass is going to look half-empty. You will not feel fully alive and vibrant. Your body, your brain, and your mind are not going to be functioning anywhere close to 100 percent.

We do so much to improve ourselves and our lives. We go to school, get the right job, work hard, read self-help books, attend workshops and seminars, study spiritual practices, go to therapy, experiment with diet and exercise fads, and endlessly tinker with our minds and bodies under the guise of "biohacking." But we never think to tap into the very thing that is the source of our bodies, our minds, and life itself.

The problem we often encounter in our self-improvement efforts is the fact that to make changes in any aspect of our lives requires a certain amount of energy to begin with. The bigger the change you want, the more energy you will need! To change anything—from your diet to your workout habits to your attitude and mind-set to your career—requires resilience, stamina, commitment, initiative, and endurance. All these words are simply descriptions of a state we can characterize as being fully charged with energy. If we don't have energy, we don't have any of these qualities. Instead, when we're low on energy, we use words like *stuck, unmotivated, unproductive, ineffective, hesitant, burned out*, and *overwhelmed*. We don't have the energy to get past our old ways of thinking and doing, so the brain keeps defaulting to what's easy and comfortable. What I'm starting to get at here is the idea that the positive qualities and positive states of mind that have served you in your life are connected with a state of *high vital force*, whereas the negative qualities that have caused you to struggle are connected with a state of *low vital force*.

Our body-mind complex is basically a rechargeable battery. We've taken this for granted, and we haven't learned to use it to improve our lives. We recharge ourselves in the obvious ways—through food, sleep, and exercise, and artificially through the use of stimulants—but we've never learned how to increase our access to the unlimited source of energy within that is keeping us alive in every moment. Let's take a closer look at the critical role that this force of vitality plays on every level of who we are.

Physical Battery

We'll start with the obvious fact that your body runs on energy. You know that energy is a mechanical requirement for the movement of your body. The body is not only chemical but electrical, and energy is what fuels any physical activity, from sitting to walking to blinking to breathing to metabolizing food to building muscle and growing physically. It's what enables your body to engage in all of its internal and external functions.

Most of us have been led to believe that the energy that fuels our system comes from three sources: food, sleep, and exercise. When you eat, it gives you not only calories and nutrients but electrical energy. It provides fuel for your mitochondria, the "brains" of your cells. When you sleep, your body temporarily goes into "rest" mode and replenishes its energy reserves. And when you exercise, the physical activity triggers a release of chemicals that brings a jolt of energy. But notice that there's a limit to how much you can energize yourself with food, sleep, and exercise alone. Eat too much, or eat the wrong foods, and you'll feel more tired and depleted. Sleep too many hours, and you'll be groggy and dull. Exercise too aggressively, and you'll barely have the energy to move. And, of course, if you don't have time to sleep or go to the gym or eat properly, then that much less energy is available to your body to do all it has to do.

In fact, food, sleep, and exercise are not the only way to recharge the system. They're not even the most efficient way. You drink your green juice, you go to the gym and sleep eight hours a night, and yet you still feel tired and run down, or maybe just not functioning at your highest capacity. That's because you're not generating enough energy to replenish the whole system, which also includes your *mind.*

Mental Battery

It's not just the body that requires energy to function optimally. Your mind also requires energy to fuel its constant activity. The number of activities the mind performs on a daily basis is even greater than the body. To have any thought requires energy. To perceive, to be alert, to be mindful, to formulate ideas, to make decisions or judgments, to strategize or analyze, to recall information—it's all electrical activity that requires an incredible amount of fuel. We've all experienced the way our cognitive functions fail us when we're tired. When our vital energy is low or not available, our minds stop working properly.

> *A busy mind is the biggest vital energy hog of all. It's a monster machine that burns up fuel like there's no tomorrow.*

When you say that you're feeling tired and run down, ask yourself what *part* of you is tired. Ninety-nine percent of the time, it's the mind, not the body, that's exhausted. We work the body-mind system during the day, and we refuel the body with food, sleep, and exercise, but it's not enough to recharge the mind. We almost never get a break from mental activity. Even when we're sleeping, the mind is still going, replaying the worries and anxieties of the day.

A busy mind is the biggest vital energy hog of all. We'll be exploring in depth the many ways that a runaway thinking mind drains our energy in Part II. For now, it's enough to know that this computer that we call "mind" is constantly running, and just like any other computer, it runs on battery power.

James Kozloski, a well-known computer neuroscientist, states, "The brain consumes a great amount of energy doing nothing." If that's true of every brain to begin with, imagine how much *more* energy is consumed by a brain that's spinning in doubts, judgments, frustrations, and endless rumination. Your brain consumes more fuel than every other part of your mind-body complex combined! It is engaged at every moment in thinking, thinking, thinking, planning, planning, planning, worrying, worrying, worrying. It doesn't shut up. You can't get it to stop thinking, no matter what you do. The mind is running even when there's no reason for it to be. It's a monster machine that burns up fuel like there's no tomorrow, and it needs to be plugged into a power source on a daily, or at least regular, basis. The more drained you feel in life, the more urgently you need to address what's going on inside your own head. This is the difference between being alive and walking around as if you are asleep in life.

How does your mind operate when you're exhausted? One of the first things that happens is that your perception becomes negative. Then your thoughts become negative. Over time, your beliefs about yourself and others become negative. Your mind goes into stress mode. You become less fluid and adaptable, less willing, more cranky, and often more adamant, fixed, and rigid in your beliefs. The lower your mental energy, the less room you have for the unexpected and the more you want things to be comfortably predictable. You need things to go "your way." You react rather than respond to situations. Your willingness to shift gears and collaborate screeches to a halt.

To challenge your own assumptions and beliefs, to look at things from a new perspective, to *respond* rather than *react* to a situation, requires mental space, some empty room in the mind. Mental space is just another way of saying "available energy." If you are fully charged, you're more patient, willing, agile, cooperative, and available to change your mind and approach as the situation requires. Your mind is more "reasonable." If you're not fully charged, your mind gets stuck in old ways of doing things.

That's when you end up in therapy or coaching, spending huge amounts of time, money, and energy trying to change your own stubborn point of view.

A depleted mind has little room to expand and let something new come in. It's like when your laptop's hard drive is full and it becomes slow, unpredictable, and prone to crashes. You move further and further away from operating in a state of present-moment awareness, in a state of "flow"—the most powerful state of mind that there is. Presence, awareness, mindfulness, flow: these qualities are all a result of high vital force on a mental level. Like computers, when our batteries are charged, we notice that there is less chatter in the mind, without us "trying" to be mindful or present. Naturally and effortlessly, we turn off the thinking mind and turn on the power of our deeper awareness, intuition, insight, and clarity.

If you want your mind to not only get you through the day but reach a state of peak performance, eating healthy, exercising, and sleeping well may not be enough. If you want to be totally focused, alert, sharp, and efficient, you will need a steady, stable fuel supply to the brain. In addition, you'll need to determine what it is that's consuming all your mental battery power. You need to see what programs are running and what files are open in the background of your mind that you don't need at the moment. Then you need to learn how to shut down the unnecessary files that are using up your energy.

The thing to remember is this: it is your mind more than anything else that determines the quality of your life, and it is your energy more than anything else that determines the state of your mind. This connection between mind, energy, and quality of life is one of the most important secrets of the Vedic tradition, and one of the most poorly understood. It's arguably the single most important key to thriving in life. That's why we're going to be talking about the mind so much in this book. If you want to increase your energy or enhance your power and positivity, the first place to look is at your own mind.

Emotional Battery

On any given day, in any given situation, you are experiencing a wide range of emotions, both positive and negative. You may not have stopped to think about it, but to feel these emotions also requires a lot of energy. To have, express, or experience any emotion (yes, even positive!) uses up battery power. Guess what? Negative emotions—as you've probably felt on many occasions—require and use up a *huge* amount of vital power. The more intense the emotion, the more energy it takes to move through it and step out of it. That's why you feel so tired, unmotivated, and stuck when you're depressed, sad, or anxious. All of your energy is going toward processing and "dealing" with that emotion.

But your emotions don't just use up energy. They can also generate and increase energy. Positive emotions give us a surge of vitality in the form of enthusiasm, joy, gratitude, love, contentment, and excitement. However, to experience the positive emotion, we need some energy to begin with. It's hard to feel happy, grateful, or excited when you're exhausted, isn't it? To laugh and live and love requires energy. If we're running low on energy, the most beautiful thing goes unnoticed or the most amazing gift can't be appreciated. Without sufficient energy, you are existing rather than really being alive—*alive* meaning able to experience the full range of human capacity, feeling, and emotion. Love, joy, happiness, gratitude, and enjoying and being present in whatever you're doing in life all require energy. When you have enough energy to be able to experience these emotions, you also get to enjoy the increase of energy that these emotions bring. It's a virtuous circle.

We need a fully charged battery to move through all of life's emotions without getting stuck in them. We'll learn in Part II how emotions wreak havoc on our energy levels and how low energy gets us more stuck in those emotions that don't serve us, sometimes for years. The more we get trapped in our negative emotions, the bigger the energy leakage and the greater the strain on the entire system.

Spiritual Battery

We also require energy to operate on a spiritual level. I'm not talking about religion; I'm talking about feeling connected to the whole, having a sense of fulfillment, meaning, and purpose in your life. I'm talking about not just living on autopilot. For many of us, the best moments of our lives are when we feel really connected to life and the people around us. This sense of connection and interconnection is what I'm calling "spirituality."

When we're depleted of energy, we notice that even the people we love the most and the things that matter to us the most seem to be a burden. We get caught up in the demands and busyness of life, we put all of our focus on the physical and material, and we quickly lose the sense of valuing what really matters. It takes energy to find meaning or purpose in anything we do. When we *do* experience a moment of connection and meaning, it brings a huge surge of energy, which makes us even more fulfilled and connected. It's another virtuous circle!

Creative and Sexual Battery

Your creative energy, which includes your sexual energy and also goes beyond it, is your passion in life. In order to create and innovate, you need big energy. When energy is low, you're less inspired and passionate. You're more "in the box." You need to have more than a bare minimum of energy in your system in order to be able to appreciate music, art, literature, theater, and film, let alone create it. It doesn't matter how creative or talented you are; if your battery gets down to 10 or 20 percent, the well of inspiration is going to run dry. Whether your creative activity is sex, art, music, tech innovating, or creative thinking, low energy means that originality, excitement, and moments of breakthrough are low.

Heck, you even need a certain amount of energy just to recognize and express your sexuality or to engage in sex. If you're tired, no matter how much you want sex or how attracted you are to the person in front of you, you're going to find yourself saying, "Not tonight, honey."

As you are reading this, there's a good chance that your energy system is running close to empty and that it's impacting everything else in your life.

As you can see, your body-mind complex, on every level, is essentially a rechargeable battery. The happiest, most successful people have the most abundant energy for life—and the most abundant energy *of* life. They know how to conserve and recharge their batteries. Nikola Tesla said that everything is energy, frequency, and vibration—tap into this force of life, and you can change everything. It's not just how cars and computers operate; it's how *you* operate. You've never been taught how to recharge your batteries, aside from the very basics of food and sleep. That's all that most of us know, but as we'll learn, there are much easier and more powerful ways.

Running on Empty

As you are reading this, there's a good chance that your energy system is running close to empty and that it's impacting everything else in your life. When you are exhausted, tired, stressed out, impatient, dull, unmotivated, distracted, or burned out, your brain is sending you a clear message: YOU ARE OUT OF FUEL! Your battery is dangerously low.

The one thing I've observed over the past 30 years in my work is that most people spend the majority of their lives living in a state of personal energy crisis. They are stuck in permanent survival mode with barely enough fuel to make it through the day. That's like hoping your smartphone will last for another eight hours when your battery is at 10 percent and there's no charger in sight. You can get by this way for a short period of time, but you will eventually burn out. We add caffeine, stimulants, and adrenaline on top of a depleted system to keep us going for a little bit longer. It might even feel like real energy, but in the long run, it's only depleting your inner energy reserves even more. Before long, your system will crash.

Your energy levels have a profound effect on the way you think, the way you feel, and the way you act, which, in turn, affects the way you move through the world and experience your life. Everything you do is infused with energy, and the state of your life will reflect the state of your energy. If you're alive and vibrant, then your life, your relationships, your business will be dynamic, radiant, and exciting. But if you're dull and drained, life becomes lukewarm. If I were to state the most precious lesson I have learned through the years, it's that where you are not thriving in life, there is always a lack of energy . . . always.

There was a time in your life when you had more energy than you knew what to do with. If you observe any child, you'll remember how much energy and vitality you had when *you* were young. Take a look at a child's face: it's full of mojo. You can see it in children's eyes, in their smiles, and hear it in their infectious laughter. You can feel it in the bounce of their movements. You know from experience that the amount of vital energy a child has—the amount of energy YOU once had—is far greater than any adult in the room. One child has enough power to wipe out all the adults in the family. You can hear the power of this innate energy in the simple, effortless gurgle of a baby that fills an entire room. The scream of a little kid is powerful enough to bring the house down! Just imagine what you could do in your life with this kind of raw power.

Toddlers barely eat more than mashed carrots and milk, and they certainly don't walk 10,000 steps a day. They don't have drugs, protein shakes, Red Bull, or Starbucks—just plenty of rest and an abundance of this power called "source energy," or vital force. Once upon a time, we all had this power. You don't need a scientist to prove this to you. You know what I'm talking about because you have personally experienced it.

You were born with all the qualities that you require to be super successful in every aspect of your life. You entered this world as a bundle of joy, enthusiasm, confidence, resilience, agility, positivity, love, acceptance, power, energy, alertness, awareness, determination, and much more. You were made up more of vitality and energy than body mass. It's a great irony that we've built multibillion-dollar industries around self-help, spirituality, therapy, and leadership development, filled with tools, books, workshops, and programs on how to cultivate the very qualities that we were born with. All of this can be boiled down to one simple key: vital force. Learn to tap into the innate power of life within you and you are home free.

A child's mind shows us what it looks like to be in a state of high vital energy on a mental level. Think back again to the way you were as a child. Any child in their natural state is full of energy. (Children who are forced to endure extreme experiences of trauma or neglect, of course, often end up with a very different set of conditions that restrict this natural vitality very early on in life. What we're talking about here is the natural state of being that every child, without exception, comes into the world with.) When you were young and full of energy, you had so much more mental agility and resilience. You could screw up horribly and then move on in a matter of moments. When you were young, your mind was filled not with fears and regrets but with a sense of freedom, expansiveness, and positivity that was most likely exponentially greater than what you experience today as an adult. You weren't stewing over yesterday or worrying about tomorrow; you were in the present moment. Your mind was unstuck, free. Even when you felt sad or angry, you could let go of those upset feelings in a matter of moments. You were full of love and positivity, bursting with creativity and enthusiasm. You didn't doubt yourself, and you weren't afraid of failing or getting rejected. Your natural state was confidence, joy, and wonder. This state of mind—the child's mind, or what we could also call a "beginner's mind"— is a direct by-product of high vital force. The opposite is also true: a vibrant, fully charged system is the natural result of a mind that's in the present moment.

It's a great irony that we've built multibillion-dollar industries around self-help, spirituality, therapy, and leadership development, filled with tools, books, workshops, and programs on how to cultivate the very qualities that we were born with.

The qualities of a child's mind, a powered-up mind—that is, life, energy, positivity, confidence, joy, awareness, resilience—all become synonymous with what I'm calling "energized." Tired, depressed, pissed off, doubting, insecure, fearful, and ineffective are just different ways of saying "depleted of energy." The intensity of the emotion indicates the level of battery charge or depletion. Clinical depression is a fully drained battery, while being head over heels in love is a fully charged battery. In between is *I'm okay. Things are fine. Same old, same old.* There's a clear link between your energy level and your ability to attract and create the life you want for yourself. Life's challenges are solved when the mind is adaptive and resilient, which is directly related to the level of energy you have. You are resilient when there's energy. When there's no energy, you get stuck.

So what happened to this innate power of yours? Where did it go? That's a bit of a misleading question, because the truth is that you are surrounded by it at all times; you're swimming in an ocean of the innate energy of life. It was never taken away from you. It's just been depleted over time, for reasons that we will discuss in detail, but that doesn't mean you can't refuel to full capacity again. Vital energy is a renewable resource—you just have to learn how to connect to it, replenish it, and keep from depleting it again.

If the science is important to you, don't worry. We'll begin to explore this in the coming chapters. But for now, I want you to begin by taking the time to actively notice what happens to your health, your ability to be focused and present, your performance at work, and the quality of your relationships when you're in a state of high versus low energy. This is important. Your own experience will act as a trusted guide as you explore deeper levels of your own innate life force.

Tapping the Source

To really supercharge our mind-body complex and therefore our lives, we need to tap into a limitless source of energy, one that's bigger than supplements and exercise regimes. We are floating at every moment in a field of this power called "life force," vital force, *Shakti*—what we might think of as "source energy." It's a field, a force of positivity itself. We just don't know how to tap into it, and we haven't really discovered what drains it. If we could figure that out, then whatever we're doing, we could do it better, stronger, and faster. We would not only do what we have to do but also everything that we *want* to do.

This innate source of energy, the positivity that we are born with, is within us and all around us. There are simple ways to tap into it. This is where the ancient Vedic tradition of India and its thousands of years of wisdom and practice will act as our guide. The West gave the world electricity, the light bulb, the energy to power the activities of our external world. The East taught us how to light up our own inner world, giving us tools to ignite and sustain the electricity within.

The ancient Vedic tradition is what I like to call the original positive psychology. It offers thousands of powerful tools to harness our life energy to manage our minds, emotions, and spirit.

In this book, we'll examine three powerful methodologies to directly tap into the power of source energy, intelligence, and positivity.

1. Breath and its connection to our thoughts and emotions—a way to effortlessly reduce stress and to be dynamic in life with a mind that is calm, present, and joyful.

2. "Effortless meditation" and its impact on letting go of trauma and old thought patterns—to help us live from a state of positivity, clarity, and high energy.

3. Mind-set shifts—to become aware of how we're operating and begin to rewire our minds.

We will explore how these three methodologies not only give us energy but also become the platform from which we co-create the vision, dreams, and life we want.

The West gave the world electricity, the light bulb, the energy to power the activities of our external world. The East taught us how to light up our own inner world.

Please keep in mind that the work we're doing here is not about self-improvement, it's about self-realization. People often make the mistake of classifying my work as a kind of self-help, which it is not. The whole concept of self-help suggests that there's something to fix, that something is wrong with the way we are. What I believe—and what the Vedic tradition teaches—is that we weren't born flawed. We were born complete: powerful, connected, joyful, vibrant, and creative. Our positivity is our essence, and that never leaves us. As we made the journey into and through adulthood, life's challenges, losses, and setbacks drained our energy and drew a veil over the perfection of who we really are. The more exhausted we get, the further we move away from our center and the power we were born with. But that veil is just a cover. It can be removed.

I'd like you to just consider the idea that you were born with the very qualities you want in life. This is the great cosmic joke: We spend a lifetime of effort and resources in order to fix and improve ourselves, only to discover we've had what we wanted all along. What we don't realize is that this source energy is the way to reboot our entire system. When we do, then we naturally, easily, and effortlessly regain those qualities that we had as children—those qualities that we so need to navigate through the chaos and the challenges of life.

The goal of every self-help and spiritual technique is to get you back to that place, back to those qualities. I believe that the best answer lies in enhancing the vital energy that you were born with. That's all you need to do! Then the energy naturally goes where it's needed, and it manifests in the things that you want to cultivate in yourself and create in your life. It's a very natural and organic process—which is why you will hear me so often use the word *effortless*. In this book, you'll learn to connect and tap into that energy, and also how to harness it so that you release what holds you back. Even holding things back takes energy! The only difference is that you're using the energy against yourself instead of channeling it constructively. It takes a lot of energy to hesitate, to hold yourself back, to resist and avoid. This same energy could be used to propel you forward.

To dream big, you need big energy. To live big, you need big energy. This is the effortless road to transforming any aspect of your life. It's the easier way. Plug into source power, connect to it, and co-create the life you want and deserve.

CHAPTER 2

Beyond Belief

When I first started exploring this idea of energy back in 1989, it was completely by accident. It wasn't something I was looking for. At the time, I had no interest whatsoever in spirituality or consciousness or Indian gurus. As you know, I was a pragmatic, left-brained lawyer (a federal prosecutor, no less), which meant that my whole life, my entire way of thinking, was about facts, evidence, achievement, and success. I only believed in what I could see or touch, and I certainly had no time to waste on empty theories with no relevance to my life. All this "love and light" New Age talk of oneness and elevating consciousness was not for real life. This touchy-feely stuff was ridiculous in my mind, and so were the people who believed in it.

People think that everyone in India meditates and does yoga and is so spiritual. I'm sorry to be the one to burst the bubble, but it's just not true. In modern India, yoga and meditation are often thought of as something from the old world, and many people tend to fight them. They're seen as the old-fashioned way of doing things. Yoga didn't even have a revival in India until after it became popular in the West! So, like most other Indians I know, I pooh-poohed all of that spiritual stuff.

I never would have ended up at Sri Sri's lecture had the hand of the universe not intervened to push me there. My father had just called me with yet another marriage prospect when I saw a magazine, pages wrinkled and stained with coffee, lying on the floor. I was picking it up to throw it away when I saw a small ad for an event with Pandit Ravi Shankar, Vedic master. Thinking it was the well-known sitar player, I called the organizers to reserve a seat. I didn't yet feel completely at home in L.A., and I was hoping that I might meet some people at this supposed sitar concert and connect with other members of the Indian community. I thought that meeting someone Indian on my own would be a happy compromise with my parents.

I had no idea what the Vedic system meant when I read the ad. I thought it was a type of classical music. When I saw the words "enlightened master," I thought it was just a fancy way of saying that he was an expert. As soon as I walked into the hall, though, I sensed that something was off. It didn't look like any concert I'd ever been to. There were no amps or microphones on the stage, just a folding chair and a vase of flowers. The audience was full of people wearing beads, flowing skirts, and pajama-style pants instead of "regular" clothes, floating around like they didn't have a care in the world and insisting on giving unwanted hugs. *Wow,* I thought to myself, *this is all that's left of this famous musician's following? Just a bunch of hippies who are into Eastern music?* When Sri Sri finally came onstage and sat down in the chair next to the flowers, it was too late to leave. And I was at least curious. That was the one thing I had going for me. Since I had gone all the way there, paid for parking, walked into the building, and taken a seat, I decided to stay.

I had no idea what the Vedic system meant when I read the ad. I thought it was a type of classical music.

Enlightened or not, I was utterly unimpressed with this so-called master. In hindsight, it was the level of stillness and peace radiating from his presence, energy, and voice that put me off at first. I couldn't wrap my head around it. I had never encountered such depth of silence and gentleness before. Funny how we are conditioned to associate value, worth, and success with hard work, effort, and authority. Sri Sri had no assertiveness, no push, no effort, yet he was clear, firm, and present.

I spent most of the lecture rolling my eyes and silently criticizing everything he was saying in my mind. *If his ideas are really so great*, I wondered, *then why isn't he teaching them back in India? There are a billion people there who need help too. I bet he's a charlatan. This is all bullshit* . . . And on and on I went. The ideas felt cheesy and sentimental, and the people in the audience nodding along enthusiastically were ridiculous by my standards—certainly not the kind of person I aspired to become or to be around. I couldn't stop thinking, *These people need to get a job.*

As the lecture went on, my internal dialogue only grew louder. *What is this stuff? This is nice for Sunday church maybe, but it has nothing to do with my life.* I really thought it was all nonsense. This airy-fairy, woo-woo philosophy felt like it belonged somewhere up in the clouds, far away from real life down here on planet Earth. I couldn't connect it to my own life in Santa Monica and the DA's office, where I was dealing with criminals and fighting for prison sentences every day. As Sri Sri discussed the nature of the mind, telling us about how our fixed and limited mind-sets block us from experiencing the flow of life, I became disgruntled and argumentative inside. I didn't mean to be judgmental; I just had never been exposed to the idea of mind, emotion, and my own inner landscape being the driving force of my life, so I wasn't buying any of it.

You have to understand that at that point in my life, working in the incredibly combative environment of the DA's office, I spent my days fighting in court. I had learned to always question people's motives and to always watch my back to make sure I wasn't being fooled. I was dealing with violent crimes, drug offenses, and murder on a daily basis. I was dealing with witnesses who kept changing their stories. Turning off my skeptical brain just wasn't an option for me. Actually, it had never even occurred to me that you could turn off your busy mind—though I was about to experience it for myself in the days ahead.

In spite of the noise in my head during the lecture, I went back and joined a weekend course. Unsurprisingly, the guru picked up on my hostile energy. At the end of the course, he looked straight at me, leaned forward in his chair, and said something I'd never forget. "Look," he told me, "you've been doing things *your way* for your entire life. If that's working for you, great—but then again, if it was working, you wouldn't be here right now. If something isn't working, you're going to have to change it, aren't you? Why don't you try this at home for 40 days and let your own experience tell you if it's working or not? If it doesn't work, you can drop it. If it does work, continue and see what it can do for your life."

This struck me as a fair deal. As a lawyer, I knew the value of evidence. I realized that I was an adult, I called myself an independent thinker, and I should be able to make my own decisions based on my own experience. Using that logic, I decided to accept Sri Sri's challenge to use the tools from the course for 40 days. As it turned out, I didn't have to wait 40 days to see the difference. After that first weekend, I went to the office on Monday and suddenly found myself operating in a total state of what's often called *flow*. All that extra white noise in my head that was always there, the usual static of worries, anxieties, and judgments, was almost entirely gone. I can only describe it as being "in the zone." Somehow everything was pouring through me, rather than me pushing and forcing and trying to control it. And that was just Monday!

Everything felt somehow different. I was more joyful and full of energy. I could do more in less time. *This is crazy*, I thought. *What did that course do to me?* I was working smarter and faster, not harder. As my mind's resistance and limiting beliefs broke down, I started moving into the flow of life, and things started coming to me. The more I embraced this flow, the more seemed to arrive in my life, as if pulled by a magnet: opportunities, new collaborations, synchronicities, help from unexpected sources. I even got a job offer from a private law firm with a salary of $250,000 and the potential for a partnership in two years. I didn't have to initiate any of it—it just came on its own. The right people showed up at the right time. When I needed something, the help was there. It was like nothing I'd ever experienced before.

Almost 30 years later, I'd like to say to you what Sri Sri said to me: *Just try it.* Explore a different way of seeing, a different way of being, and a set of practices that can help you get there. You don't even have to try it for 40 days if you don't want to, although I'd recommend it. Just try on the ideas and practices in this book for the duration of time that you're reading it. Be open. Set aside your beliefs for the moment and play around with a bigger way of seeing yourself and the world. Do you really have anything to lose? The time that you "lose" doing the practices will be made up tenfold in the energy you gain. My advice to you is to be scientific about it, conduct an experiment on yourself, and see what happens. This is what real science is, after all. It's what we call "the proof in the pudding."

Please, question everything you find in these pages! Stay curious. Be smart, and by "smart," I mean letting your experience speak for itself. You'll find the answers for yourself by testing out these ideas and tools and applying them in your own life. What you will notice is that things will start shifting in a very short span of time—you'll start to feel it within moments and see results in a matter of a few days. That's the real power of these ideas and techniques: they are able to almost instantly transform the way you perceive the world in front of you. That's why they have stood the test of time for thousands of years. What we're talking about isn't mysticism; it's a very practical philosophy for living your highest potential.

Please, question everything you find in
these pages! Stay curious. You'll find
the answers for yourself.

I am asking you to explore the idea—just for now—that we live in a world of limitless energy, intelligence, and possibilities. I'm also asking you to consider the idea that this unlimited energy, intelligence, and potentiality lies within you and is accessible to you. Again, I'm not asking you to believe in what I'm saying; I'm asking you to explore it through your own experience. *Belief* refers to accepting something without proof, which goes against all my training in life. Proof based on another person's standards is also not enough. What's proven today is often disproven tomorrow. The best proof is your own experience, your own search inside yourself. Let that be your guide in exploring the power of energy in your life.

You may have to put your disbelief aside, roll up your sleeves, and decide to go for it in order to find that extra edge that may be missing in your life. If you want a life that's beyond what you're living right now, then you're going to have to do things you've never done before. That means being willing to be a beginner, to try something new and approach it with an open mind. I say this to you as a fellow traveler in the journey of life and as a teacher who has personally seen hundreds of thousands of lives transformed as a result of these ancient technologies, the wisdom and techniques in this book.

The Power within and around You

Let's take a closer look at what the Vedic tradition has to say about this unlimited energy that we're talking about—this energy that manifests in the many ways we discussed in the last chapter.

In Vedanta, vital force or life energy is sometimes called *Shakti*, or, when embodied, *prana*. In yogic traditions, *Shakti* is the original creative force from which all things arise (for this reason, it's also called "source energy"). It is the primordial cosmic power that moves everything in the universe, the invisible principle that governs all things. It's unseen, but it drives every aspect of life. This energy is all around us, and it's also inside of us. It is this source that energizes our physical, mental, emotional, spiritual, sexual, and creative battery.

Shakti isn't some impersonal, inanimate, mechanical force, nor is it some god to be worshipped. It's intelligent and conscious, and it's also loving and nurturing. *Shakti* is understood as the feminine principle of the world we perceive through our senses. I'll explain a bit later what I mean by "feminine principle," but what's important for you to know right now is that *this is a force that you can connect with, call upon, and enter into a relationship with.* It's a force that you can access in order to enhance your life. The liberation of this potent feminine creative energy within ourselves—so that we can be fully vital and alive—is what we're going for here. Keep an open mind. We're charting a new path based on timeless wisdom and ancient mystical tools, and that path is going to take us deep into the unknown.

If you enter into a relationship with this energy, it moves you, it fuels you, and it serves you. It's a fiercely loving, nourishing power. It's healing and regenerative. You may not be a believer in this life force or in any kind of universal consciousness, but I'm sure you're aware of the many discussions going on within the scientific community about energy and consciousness, about the nature of our quantum reality. Philosophers and mystics have been discussing this for eons, and today, neuroscientists and physicists are joining the conversation. If the language of spirituality doesn't work for you, don't get hung up on it. Know that brilliant minds like Albert Einstein, Nikola Tesla, and Max Planck engaged in endless discussion and experimentation around the nature of this mysterious life force—the substance underlying all of reality—and the field of intelligence that surrounds us. They knew that we move in this dynamic, interconnected field of energy like fish in water, even if they weren't yet able to prove it. For now, suffice it to say that just because you can't see this energy or "prove" it scientifically doesn't mean that it doesn't exist. Of course, that also doesn't mean that it *does* exist, so we'll allow the question to remain open. In the end, your experience, your results, and your self-study are the best proof for you.

> *We have to discover how our own energy system*
> *works and how to enhance the energy of life*
> *that we're born with. Without this energy,*
> *this machine that is you won't even turn on,*
> *much less operate at peak performance.*

Without energy, as we've discussed, we are slow and sluggish. Pushing and pulling with willpower to get through the day is not an effective or lasting solution. We have to discover how our own energy system works and how to enhance the energy of life that we're born with. Without this energy, this machine that is *you* won't even turn on, much less operate at peak performance. Low energy cripples our minds by creating a perception of *I can't, it's too much,* and thus a sense of resistance. This life energy helps us function more optimally, but at the same time, it also does something much deeper. Accessing the source of energy within ourselves allows us to tap into the flow of life: the place where all creation and manifestation occurs.

The Force of Life

> *All matter originates and exists only by virtue of a force. . . .*
> *We must assume behind this force the existence of a conscious*
> *and intelligent Mind. This Mind is the matrix of all matter.*
>
> — MAX PLANCK, QUANTUM PHYSICIST AND NOBEL LAUREATE

Throughout this book, I'll be using the terms *innate energy, life energy, life force, vital force, source energy,* and *Shakti* interchangeably, so keep in mind that they all mean the same thing. The Vedic tradition talks a lot about this concept of vital force, but it's not an idea that exists only in India. Almost every culture has its own language for describing this universal energy that animates all living things and connects us in a dynamic web of life. In Chinese medicine, it's called *qi,* the life-giving energy that underlies the human system and all of nature. The Chinese described qi as the force that animates life, a kind of nonmaterial essence that manifests in all matter. The ancient Greeks knew this source energy as *pneuma* (translated as "breath," "spirit," or "soul"), or what the philosopher Zeno called the "creative fire." *Pneuma* was thought of as the active principle organizing the individual and the cosmos, the force that gives structure to matter. Even American pop culture talks about this mysterious energy of life: if you've seen *Star Wars*, you know it as *the Force*. Jedi master Obi-Wan Kenobi describes it perfectly to Luke Skywalker: "The Force is what gives a Jedi his power. It's an energy field created by all living things. It surrounds us and penetrates us; it binds the galaxy together."

We know from quantum physics that we are basically swimming in a sea of energy at all times. Even the big bang theory says that at the beginning, there was pure energy, and it exploded to create all that exists in the universe.

This field of energy that penetrates all things—made up of electrical impulses, vibrations, and frequencies—is not just empty space. It is filled with information. Vedanta says that there is energy, and there is also intelligence. The field of energy also contains an all-knowingness that the mystics call "consciousness." Sometimes the Vedic masters call it the "Big Mind," or, as Planck said, a conscious and intelligent Mind (with a capital M). This consciousness is also known in Vedanta as *Shiva*, the masculine element. According to the Vedas, the fundamental unifying force upon which everything is built is this field of energy and intelligence. The field has both dynamic energy (*Shakti*) and pure awareness or consciousness (*Shiva*). They are two sides of the same coin: the feminine and the masculine, the seen and the unseen, the manifested and the unmanifested, the movement and the stillness, the actuality and the potentiality. Consciousness or intelligence by itself is dormant, but when activated, it becomes energy. Energy can then remain in a subtle, or unseen, state, or if it becomes dense enough, it can convert itself into matter. That's the short story of how our own unseen intentions go from thought forms to manifested material reality.

The sages say that the field contains within it all information, a record of everything that has ever occurred and will ever occur. To tap into this field of information or wisdom—the source of all clarity, intuition, insights, and "aha!" moments—you just need to tune your mental machinery to the right frequency. You need to clear out enough of the noise in your mind so that you can get a clear signal. The mind, like a computer using Wi-Fi, needs a strong signal to be able to download information. The tools provided in this book have been used for thousands of years as a way to do exactly that: to clear the mental debris, get the static out of the signal, and expand awareness so that the mind can tune in to a wider field of information. From that space of expanded consciousness, you can download all the potentiality of who you are. You just have to make your signal strong to connect to it. How do you do that? By enhancing your vital force, which naturally expands your consciousness to access more of this field of information. Remember, energy and innate intelligence are two sides of the same coin: raise your energy, and your consciousness will expand along with it. Expand your consciousness, and you will naturally raise your energy. This book includes tools for addressing both sides.

The Power of Prana

So where is this life force to be found in this mind-body machine that you call "me"? It's not isolated in some specific part of your brain or body. Instead, it's a *field* surrounding and interpenetrating the body. It permeates every cell of our entire being. It is the substratum of what we're made up of, along with the five elements of earth, water, fire, air, and space. We might say it's the element of aliveness or the element of thriving. It's the force that helps a flower grow from seed to full bloom, and it does the same for us—using the information encoded in our DNA to help us grow to our full potential.

---

*Energy and innate intelligence are two sides
of the same coin: raise your energy, and your
consciousness will expand along with it. Expand
your consciousness, and you will naturally
raise your energy.*

Without energy to bring it to life, physical matter is inert, dead. In the same way that water is a basic requirement of life, life cannot exist in the absence of *Shakti*. In the human system, *Shakti* flows into an embodied form as what's called *prana*, a Sanskrit word referring to the energy that powers mind, body, and spirit. This energy, which is the stimulus for all physical and cognitive functions, determines the state of functioning of the entire system. When vital energy is low, we are tired and fatigued, our mood and focus decline, and our bodies become susceptible to illness. The higher our energy levels, the more the performance of all of our faculties is heightened: the body becomes healthier, the mind and intellect become quick and sharp, our mood is elevated, and on and on. Life energy powers every part of the machine—all of you.

The field of electromagnetic energy around the body is sometimes called the "human biofield," and the energy itself is sometimes referred to by scientists as "bioenergy" or "bioplasma." As we've said, our individual energetic biofield is part of this larger field of energy that permeates and surrounds us. This is scientific in the fullest sense of the word. Even researchers at universities like Harvard, Princeton, and Yale have studied this field of energy and the way it operates in peer-reviewed, double-blind studies and randomized controlled trials. Many alternative healing modalities that have now been studied scientifically—from acupuncture to Reiki to qigong to sound therapy—work by directing and strengthening the flow of life energy in and around the body.

As we've said, this energy takes on an infinite variety of different manifestations in our lives depending on the medium through which it is flowing and expressing itself. You can't see it, but you know it well. Vital force can take the form of physical energy: movement and motion, the "get-up-and-go," that fire under your ass when you really need to get something done. It's the power that makes things go and keeps them going. On a mental and emotional level, it's passion and motivation, the mojo, the *juice*, the gusto. It's that extra zest, an indescribable "special something." In business and work, it shows up as initiative and risk-taking, the force that propels innovation, growth and evolution, resilience and agility. On another level, it's your most potent creative and sexual energy—the force that brings new life, whether in the form of ideas or embryos. On a spiritual level, it's that deeper awareness and connection to the whole of life. When the flow of life energy is strong and clear, you experience a state of health and harmony in the body. This vitality enlivens every cell of your being.

In the Vedic system, harnessing the energy of life is the key to success, the key to happiness, the key to being present, and the key to feeling connected to the whole. If you could find a way to bottle and sell this energy, you'd be a billionaire. Why? Because it's that extra *oomph* that we're all looking for. It's our mojo! It's the secret sauce for all of life.

Let's look a little closer at some of the ways that operating from a place of high energy and potentiality fuels success.

The Secret Sauce

If you asked my husband, he'd probably say the secret sauce for all of life is butter. Leaving that aside, what I'm calling the "secret sauce" is this certain magic quality we sense in people who are full of life force. We feel it immediately, and we're attracted to it, even if we can't explain exactly why. We're drawn to people who are passionate, dynamic, successful, full of joy and confidence—those who are animated by the power of life itself. It's in a person's *vibe*. We feel it in that person who lights up the room as soon as they walk in. We can catch a glimpse of it in someone's eyes and in their smile. It's not just luck or good genes, it's the energy of life.

I love Tony Robbins as an example of the power of this force. He is so overflowing with life energy that he's become a true force of nature. There's an undeniable larger-than-life quality to him, a power and magnetism that's propelled him to unthinkable success. The man is a machine: he runs a handful of companies valued at billions of dollars, coaches the most successful people in the world, and spends months of the year at workshops where he's onstage for 12 hours straight, guiding thousands of people through personal breakthroughs. He's jumping around, he's getting everyone hyped up, he's yelling, he's making people laugh and cry. He goes, goes, goes, but where is his focus? It's not externalized. His "business," what he does for a living, inherently and naturally requires that he put his attention *inside* . . . and as a result, he naturally taps into and generates huge amounts of this innate source energy we're talking about. That's what fuels him and everyone in his audience for 12 hours at a time. He has a lot of energy projecting out into the world, but his focus is on moving the furniture around in the internal space so that he can act from a place of clarity and strength. He's changing his mental habits and inspiring others to do the same in order to create internal power. This inner energy is something he cultivates deliberately. In fact, if you go to a Tony Robbins Unleash the Power Within or Date with Destiny event, you'll notice that he actually uses certain breathing exercises derived from the Vedic techniques we'll be discussing in this book as an "energy break" to keep his audience engaged.

High vital force also manifests as leadership and star power. It enhances soft skills like authenticity, sincerity, compassion, and collaboration from the inside out—not as a strategic, manipulated behavior but as a genuine expression of who we are. It's what gives leaders the ability to inspire others and start a movement. If you look at great historical figures like Gandhi, Martin Luther King, and Nelson Mandela, you can see this in action. There's a kind of juice in their system that comes through when they speak, expressing itself in a certain fluctuation and tone in the voice. With one little line, "I have a dream," Martin Luther King conveyed so much emotion and energy. *That* is life force. That's the same innate power you have within you.

Defying Your Limits

I've led countless workshops and seminars for business leaders and worked with many top executives, and I can tell you with certainty that leadership is never about the résumé. It's always about the indescribable. It's about going beyond the boundaries of your own conditioning and acting from the core of your being, from your most natural state. Generally, any person who becomes a true leader—whether in their own family or community, in business or art, or in government—is someone who has reached into a place within themselves that is beyond what they were taught and conditioned to believe is possible.

Leaders' potentiality is not contained in what they know about themselves or what they've seen around them. Leadership potentiality is when they see, and then leap, "outside the box." The box is our conditioned thinking, our belief systems, our limits, our ideas of "what is" based on what we see, touch, and feel. The unknown, the potentiality outside of your lowercase-*s* self, is beyond your mind's ability to see, touch, and feel. What you can measure has a limit, but you yourself are limitless. If you can dip into that unlimited space, then you start looking out of your eyes beyond what you and the things around you appear to be. Only then can you live from your greatness and inspire others to do the same.

When we're operating from BS (as in "belief systems"), we continuously minimize who we are. We reduce our identity and our capacity to something smaller than it really is. Think about it: If my goal is to achieve a certain thing, then the most I'm going to target to achieve is that thing, whether it's the business I want to create or the partner I want to attract or the home I want to buy. If what I've seen and heard throughout my pivotal early years sets a limit on something, then that limit becomes the full extent of what I will go for. That's what I mean when I say that we operate in our own limited sphere of thinking, when *who we are* is actually unlimited. Our greatness is not in achieving what we know we can achieve. If I know I can jump 10 feet, and I jump 10 feet, well then, big deal! Our greatness lies in achieving what we didn't know was possible. That means going outside of your conditioned mind. That means setting your sights higher than you know you can go—setting a goal of jumping 20 feet even though everything in you tells you that only 10 is possible.

Remember, I was trained as a lawyer! Indian, practical, pragmatic. One plus one equals two. How to propel a vision of limitless was not something I learned at home or in school. I had to leap out of the field of my mind's known possibilities and into the field of unknown possibilities.

You've heard the story of how we started Art of Living with just four teachers. After a few years of traveling and launching new centers, the four of us wanted to stay at our home center to have more time to enjoy with the master and each other. In my mind I would tell myself, *One day, we're going to have 100 teachers. Then the four of us won't have to go anywhere; the new teachers can travel for us.* From four, imagining 100 was an exponential growth leap because I had to extend my beliefs beyond the current reality of four teachers running everything. When we hit 100, my wild imagination started to say, *When we have 5,000 teachers, then we can really just hang loose and relax.* I started wanting to test the universe to see how far I could go from four! If I had stayed within the confines of my inside-the-box thinking, I could have gotten to maybe 400 at the most. But by tapping into our deepest power and potential to challenge the limits of what was possible, the four of us somehow expanded to 50,000 teachers just within India—and counting! *That* is outside of conditioned thinking.

And remember, I was trained as a lawyer! Indian, practical, pragmatic. One plus one equals two. How to propel a vision of limitless was not something I learned at home or in school. I had to leap out of the field of my mind's known possibilities and into the field of unknown possibilities. If I told you you could put in $4 million and get $40 million back, you'd doubt that it was possible. You'd say, *What do you mean? Tell me, give me the business proposition.* You'd want to see a proposal and analyze it and do your due diligence. You'd be looking at it through the lens of your limited mind to make sure that everything added up. And, of course, that's reasonable and often necessary. But it's not what true success is about. When we reach a goal that we see as within our capacity, we do not feel like it's success: it's simply that we could and we did. When we leap outside our box of possibilities, we feel as if we have arrived, we have succeeded. Leadership is what happens when you take other people out of the box with you. Those who are really successful do just that. They don't do something just because it's reasonable. They are "mad" in nature—meaning operating outside of the norm, in the sense that the ancients spoke of as being divinely inspired.

Finding Flow

Being connected to vital force also fuels success on a practical, everyday level by fueling productivity and high performance, as I experienced so powerfully after my first workshop. If you look at monks and serious meditation practitioners, they're often eating and sleeping much less than the average person. But not only are they full of energy, they are also capable of seemingly impossible mental feats. That's because they're living *in the flow of life.* Talk to enough successful people, and you'll find that most of them have strategies that they use for enhancing their internal energy and accessing what we call "flow states." We know that a state of flow—where self-consciousness is transcended and we become one with whatever we're doing— is key to creativity, insight, and sustained focus. It's also one of the best ways to enhance your energy, because when you're in a state of flow, you're tapped into the source of energy itself, and you're being fueled by that energy. It's an energy that never runs dry. It's infinitely replenishable.

It shouldn't come as much of a surprise, then, that productivity-obsessed Silicon Valley has gotten in on the energy secret. Entrepreneur, venture capitalist, and Bulletproof CEO Dave Asprey created a billion-dollar empire around the idea of "biohacking" one's physiology for energy and peak performance, and he draws on many of the ancient tools of Vedanta in this quest for self-optimization. Asprey wrote on his blog that he practiced Art of Living breathing techniques (the same ones I learned from Sri Sri on the night of the "concert") daily for five years as a way to hack his nervous system. "I met a group of overwhelmingly successful entrepreneurs once a week on Saturday morning at 7 A.M. to practice it together," he wrote. "It's a simple, repeatable method used by 25 million people worldwide. . . . It works."

In my past life as a prosecutor, I already had a high-performing life before I found these tools. I was managing a busy schedule and a demanding workload, even though I woke up tired in the morning and I didn't know why. I could make it through the day without thinking there was anything wrong, but when I started consciously cultivating my energy, it opened up another world. Suddenly I was doing the same things I had been doing before—same food, same exercise, same job, same friends—but with a sense of gusto. I was always ready to go for it. That's the feeling that came into my system. When I realized how my mind was draining me and cutting me off from the flow of life, and I learned these tools to replenish my life force, I could suddenly get things done in a fraction of the time. I didn't have to hype myself up to go to work or get things done; I was just naturally in a dynamic, productive state. Suddenly, time wasn't a problem anymore. I stopped needing 9 or 10 hours of sleep to feel fully rested. I'm sleeping less and leading 10-day retreats for thousands of people in the U.S., South America,

Europe, or India and then traveling across the globe to lead another retreat. It's work that requires tremendous output.

I'm often asked how I keep up with all the demands in my life. I fly around the globe regularly, I teach hundreds of people in any given week, I lecture to huge audiences, and I spend many hours a day listening to people's questions and problems, which requires my full attention and care. And trust me, people don't usually come to me to tell me about the great things in their lives. They come to share their challenges and struggles, whether it's their aging parents, their health, their finances, or their depression. I may not have an answer, but it's the attention and tools I give them that allow them to go home feeling uplifted and resilient, with this confidence that they can handle the challenge, whatever it is. What I can tell you is that it's not really coming from me so much as it's the life force that they increase in themselves that transforms them.

The truth is that my relationship to the all-connected creative force of life is my secret weapon. Not always, but much of the time, it's not really me who is doing the work. There's something working through me. I recently gave a lengthy talk at PayPal, and I didn't even know what the topic was until I showed up. Being present is the best preparation for anything. I walked into PayPal and asked them, "What are we talking about today?" and I moved with it. To me, it doesn't really matter what the work is. I show up, I'm present, and I allow myself to be an instrument for something greater. I call on my relationship with *Shakti,* with this energy that allows things to happen organically. When I'm in the flow of the moment, the energy is near limitless. When I'm really effective, when I'm at my most clear, I know that I'm tapped into something beyond my own ego, talents, or intellect. I'm allowing myself to become a useful instrument for what wants and needs to happen. In these moments, the surge of energy, creativity, and clear intelligence that I experience is something I can't even put into words.

I share my own experience to show what's available to each and every one of us. This isn't something foreign or inaccessible;

you've experienced it before. If you look back at your life, I am willing to bet that you can think of at least a few of these moments of total clarity and connection. You're so in the moment that things come out of you that you never could have planned for. Maybe it was a time that you lost yourself in the creative process, or got up on stage and gave the talk of your life, or a moment of joy when you were completely in love or totally present to the beauty of nature. Perhaps it was a moment of utter clarity when you were struck with the sudden awareness of *exactly* what you needed to do next. In these moments, you are tapped into something greater, and you become a vessel for the energy of creation itself to flow through. When you do this, you access a field of not only power but also pure intelligence, pure potentiality, pure consciousness.

We don't have to leave these moments up to chance. The more that you consciously engage with the life energy within yourself, the more the greater force of life will step in to help you. Moments of flow will magnify and multiply. The more you connect to this force, the more it activates the creative power within you. That's what *Shakti* is: a dynamic, creative force that is intended to manifest in the world. It literally translates to "manifested creation." We know from Einstein that energy converts itself into matter. That is what's happening here. When you connect to *Shakti*, you're connecting to your own manifesting power. You're connecting to your own nature as a creator.

If you look back at your life, I am willing to bet that you can think of at least a few of these moments of total clarity and connection. We don't have to leave these moments up to chance.

Like the Madonna in Christianity, in India we say prayers to *Devi*, the divine mother. There's a nine-day celebration every year during which this feminine energy is honored, and connecting to it is thought to be like connecting to your mother—meaning the essence of unconditional love. You honor her, and she gives you her love, care, and support. At other times you connect with your father, and he gives you his love and care and support. They both have their own unique ways to love you and give you what you need. And the more you build a relationship with the two sides that come together to create this creative and intelligent force of life, the more this power wakes up in you.

CHAPTER 3

Ancient Biohacking

Thousands of years ago, a scientist sat cross-legged beside a river. Listening to the sounds of the flowing water, he observed the ebb and flow of his own thoughts and emotions. This scientist was an expert in the mind. He had spent decades learning how it functions and how to optimize those functions, using his own mind as his laboratory. With self-observation and self-awareness as his experimental tools, he developed methods for preserving and enhancing the energy within himself that fueled and sustained all of his cognitive functions.

This scientist, also known as a *rishi*, developed the power to maximize and harness this thing he called "vital force." He discovered that the energy that gave him life and kept him alive wasn't just physical—it was also intimately connected to the state of his own mind. In fact, he observed a two-way relationship between the level of vital force in his system and the functioning of his mind, such that a change in one always triggered a change in the other. He saw that underlying the qualities he sought to cultivate in his own mind—joy, presence, vitality, calm, connectedness—was a state of high energy. When vital force was high, his mind was sharp, vibrant, and powerful. His consciousness was expanded and uplifted. Wisdom and clarity came in.

When vital force was low, the mind was ineffective. It got stuck in all kinds of things: thoughts of the past and future, negative beliefs and emotional reactions, doubts and frustrations, judgments of self and other. The more depleted the energy system, the more the mind would get caught up in thoughts and emotions that seemed to drain his energy even further. Low energy, he also noticed, was always accompanied by a contracted state of consciousness—meaning a reduced level of awareness.

This rishi, whom many called a "seer," discovered that not only could he directly impact his mental state and his thoughts by hacking his own energy system—*anyone* could impact his or her own mind and energy matrix. From the repeated findings of the self-study conducted by this rishi and many others, two important conclusions arose: (1) living optimally is a function of expanding our consciousness, and (2) when we use certain tools and methodologies to enhance our innate energy, our consciousness naturally expands.

The tools that this rishi developed for tapping into source energy were encoded in a set of sacred scriptures more than 5,000 years old known as the *Vedas*, a series of texts that includes teachings, stories, hymns, and poems on subjects ranging from neuroscience and health to physics, history, and cosmology. These texts are the original basis for the yogic and Buddhist traditions. Take a look inside the *Vedas*, and you will find a kind of operating manual for the human mind—a user's guide, if you will. It explains in detail the science of how your mind, body, and energy systems function, and how to optimize those functions. The branch of the *Vedas* that details the ancient science for understanding the mind is known as *Vedanta* (*veda* meaning "knowledge" and *anta* meaning "end of" or "culmination"). If you literally translate it, *Vedanta* means "the ultimate wisdom" as it relates to oneself: how to handle the mind, how to maximize energy, and how to be healthy in the body. Much like Buddhism, Vedanta teaches that the more you can manage your mind, the more you can change everything in life. It also provides the practical everyday tools for mind management. For the purposes of this book, the terms *Vedic*, *Vedanta*, and *yogic* may be used interchangeably.

---

*We are taking a journey to access the conscious-
ness that gives life to the mind. We're going to
the very source of thought and emotion in order
to change the way we think and feel.*

So many currently popular wellness trends—yoga, mindfulness, emotional intelligence training, performance enhancement, biohacking, and even things like hypnotherapy and
neuro-linguistic programming (NLP)—are about managing the
mind. These tools for managing thoughts are important and
valuable, but as the rishis found, there is a simpler and more
effective way—a more direct way to affect the mind without
focusing, labeling, or monitoring our thoughts and emotions
through yet more mental activity. The rishis taught us that the
most natural, effortless way to become the master of your own
mind is by raising your own fundamental vital force. Through
this thing called "vital force," we are taking a journey to access
the consciousness that gives life to the mind. We're going to the
very source of thought and emotion in order to change the way
we think and feel.

The ancient techniques of Vedanta have been around for
more than 5,000 years for a good reason: *they work.* In fact, you
probably already know and practice some of the techniques of
Vedanta, although you may not have realized that was what
you were doing. If you've ever done a downward-facing dog,
you've practiced Vedic techniques for managing the mind. In
the West, many of us haven't quite realized that yoga exercises
are techniques to not only strengthen the body but also manage
the mind. Yoga and Ayurveda, the health and nutritional
philosophy of India, are both branches of the Vedanta tradition.
The system of yoga is simply a practical methodology for what
Vedanta offers: a way to bring body, mind, breath, intellect,
memory, and ego to function at their optimum, thriving state.
When you're operating at your peak state of being, you are in
a state of *yoga*, which means to "yoke" or "unite." You connect

and harmonize all the different aspects of who you are. Now a very valid question might arise in your mind: How? How do you get to a state of yoga? That's exactly what Vedanta describes, including the traditional physical postures and exercises of hatha yoga. These techniques aren't just made up; they come from decades of methodical self-observation. Traditional hatha yoga poses involve movements that all human beings naturally make. Watch a baby for a while, and you'll see that every single yoga posture is something babies do as they're growing and developing different aspects of themselves. Babies twist into triangle pose as their livers and digestive systems develop, and they roll over into a cobra as their spines are lengthening and strengthening. A child does literally every traditional yoga posture! As adults, we can use these postures to return the body to its natural state of thriving.

Yoga is just one small part of the larger science of Vedanta. As a whole, Vedanta is a complete system for reconnecting to the source energy that gives us life and keeps us alive. While yoga has become extremely popular again today, the deeper wisdom of energy management (or "energy intelligence," as I like to call it) has gotten more lost over the years. *This* is where we must turn to recharge our minds and our selves.

These teachings are extraordinarily rich and juicy, and to this day, they are decades ahead of our most advanced sciences. Neuroscientists today study the brain to understand how thoughts and mental frameworks function, but these frameworks were understood thousands of years ago by rishis who looked at themselves and noticed how their own thoughts worked. The difference between the modern neuroscientists and the ancient scientists is that those ancient seers studied their own minds and the mechanisms of the brain, while the modern scientist studies pictures of someone else's brain. All the science that's behind what we're discovering today in brain science and psychology, the rishis already knew. We're going to take a closer look at Vedanta as a science of the mind in order to give you a better sense of where these concepts and tools originated and why they're still relevant to us today.

The Original Positive Psychology

Like the modern concept of positive psychology, Vedanta teaches us what it means to thrive as human beings. It also uses research-tested techniques that tell us exactly what we need to do in order to get there. Similarly again to positive psychology, Vedanta has always examined the mind from the point of view of health and well-being, never disease and pathology. Mindfulness, gratitude, happiness, resilience, compassion . . . all these things that positive psychology talks about have been studied for millennia, long before even the time of the Buddha or Christ.

You might be surprised at just how many of our groundbreaking modern scientific discoveries were already common knowledge to the ancients. Here's just one example: Scientists have "proved" that gratitude has the power to transform our health and well-being. Studies show that practicing gratitude positively impacts brain function, improves physical health and cardiovascular function, and increases vitality and longevity.[1] We now know that a mind-set of gratitude impacts the body on a cellular level, even altering DNA expression.[2] It brings health, it brings happiness, it brings more energy, and it even brings more life—and a *longer* life. That's great, but it's nothing new. The Vedic masters could have told you this over 5,000 years ago! They saw this when they looked inside their own minds. They knew that a certain expansive mind-set of appreciation and abundance brings health and well-being to the body, mind, emotions, and also the spirit. (More on this in Chapter 9, "Living Your Inner Superpowers.")

Consider just a handful of recent "discoveries" that can be traced back millennia to the ancient science of the Vedas:

Happiness creates success (not the other way around).

We all strive for success because we think it will make us happier, but it's been proven a thousand and one times that *happiness is what creates success*, not the other way around. In 2012, a review of 225 studies published in the journal *Psychological*

Bulletin found that achieving success doesn't necessarily lead to positive emotions and increased well-being. Instead, these studies showed that happy people seek out goals that reinforce their current state of happiness, and they're more proactive and motivated in achieving those goals.[3] In other words, they do the exact things that lead to the ultimate outcome of success. Vedanta has always said that happiness is a state of energy that leads to more positive and powerful thoughts, behaviors, and actions—and that happiness, not success, is primary.

There are three main pathways to happiness.

The rishis tell us that there are three levels of happiness: pleasure, engagement, and meaning. Martin Seligman, the father of positive psychology, talks about happiness in this same trinity![4] There's pleasure (*I bought a new car, I look good, I'm having fun, I'm out with my friends*), which is akin to the immediate gratification that Vedanta calls "sense pleasure." That's the lowest tier. It's short-lived, it comes and goes, and the more you chase after it, the emptier you feel—meaning the more you need in order to feel happy again. The next layer of happiness is engagement, being proactive and dynamic. So there's the sense-pleasure you get from watching soccer on TV, the first level, and then there's the more lasting happiness of *engaging* in a game of soccer yourself. Vedanta talks about this second level of happiness as something more than just pleasing the senses. The mind is also very active in it, and as a result, you go a little deeper and find *meaningfulness.* You might feel a deep sense of meaning, for instance, from coaching a kids' soccer team. You're engaged, but on top of that there's also a sense of camaraderie, brotherhood, and service. This brings an even more lasting happiness.

But it doesn't stop there. There's another level of happiness that Vedanta talks about, which positive psychology hasn't quite arrived at yet. At this level, you ARE happiness itself. A baby, without any particular reason, exudes joy, peace, and happiness.

The baby *is* happiness by its nature. It's a joy that is not dependent on anything external, a joy that simply radiates out from the deepest place within. Happiness is the very substance that we are made up of. It's the essence of who we are at our core. This unchanging state of happiness that you are is not dependent on anything external; it's the very nature of your consciousness. It's how we are born: as "a bundle of joy."

Meditation does a mind and body good.

How many times have you been told that meditation is good for your health? There are literally thousands of scientific studies proving that meditation can improve almost every aspect of life, including boosting positive emotions and well-being, improving physical health, increasing creativity and focus, boosting empathy and improving relationship quality, and fostering more effective leadership.[5] Again, these are all things that we've known since ancient times. Vedanta has always described meditation as a tool for bringing the mind, body, and spirit into a state of thriving.

It's important to clarify that when we talk about meditation in Vedanta, we're talking about something very different from what we think of as mindfulness practice in the Western world (more on this in Chapter 6). But suffice it to say that the benefits of meditation were well known thousands of years before modern science even came to be.

There's another level of happiness that Vedanta talks about, which positive psychology hasn't quite arrived at yet. At this level, you ARE happiness itself.

Everything is energy.

If you want to find the secrets of the universe, think in terms of energy, frequency, and vibration.

Can you guess who said these words? It wasn't some Indian guru or ancient philosopher. It was actually the physicist and engineer Nikola Tesla, a longtime student of the Vedas and a friend of the Indian spiritual teacher Swami Vivekananda. Tesla spent years trying to prove the principles of Eastern metaphysics using Western scientific methods, and he even used Sanskrit terms (including *prana*) in his descriptions of natural phenomena. Tesla wanted to prove that everything really *is* energy.

But what does that mean exactly? According to Vedic cosmology, all of life is made up of *prana* and *akasha*, or energy in movement in space. Even our bodies and minds are free-flowing biochemical and electrical energy, and scientists have shown that there is an electromagnetic field within and surrounding the body known as the *human biofield*. If that sounds familiar, it should: this is simply an ancient version of Einstein's general theory of relativity! Tesla tried his best, but it wasn't until Einstein came along with $E=mc^2$ that we could recognize the similarity to the cosmology of the rishis. Einstein proved that matter and energy were simply different manifestations of the same basic substance—what the Vedas describe, as we've learned, as an all-pervasive, unified field of consciousness.

⁓

This list could go on and on. You could spend years studying the Vedas and barely scratch the surface of the knowledge hidden in those pages. For our purposes, we want to focus on what Vedanta tells us about the mind and the tools it provides to turn off the busy thinking mind and develop what I call the "Big Mind": the peaceful, dynamic true power of our consciousness.

The Indian tradition of getting 12 years of education for your outer world and 12 years of education for your inner world is long gone. Unfortunately, today none of us spend 12 years, or even one year, learning how to deal with the noise in our heads. At some point in our adult lives, when we realize we are healthy on the outside but dying on the inside—overloaded, exhausted, or miserable—we finally agree to take responsibility for our own inner experience. We agree we have to manage our own minds. And before we learn the tools to do this, we first have to understand how this machine called "mind" functions and how it's draining all of our energy to begin with.

Part II

BRAIN

DRAIN

CHAPTER 4

A Machine Called Mind

Your human mind is the foundation for everything you think, feel, and do. It is the basis from which you achieve all that you want in life. First comes thought, then comes action, and only then come the results. Where your mind puts its awareness and attention, that is what grows in your life. It is the one thing that can transform everything, for better or for worse. If you want to excel in all that you do in your life, then you need to know how your mind functions, how to manage it, and how to apply it to the things that matter most to you. All of the objects we own come with instructions, but unfortunately, the thing we use more than anything else is missing its manual. Nowhere in life, not at home or in school, have we learned how to operate our minds efficiently and effectively.

Everything depends on the state of your mind, from your thoughts, perceptions, decisions, and judgments to figuring out what you want in life. So where do you begin? The obvious place to start is by opening up the hood of this machine called "mind" and taking a look at what's inside. You need to look at what kind of programs and inputs make it operate in a present, alert, and clear state and which ones make its functions become dull, foggy, and confused.

Let's go back to the big question that this book started with: *Who are you?* Don't get too philosophical here. I'm not talking about the Self at this point. Try to think about the question as concretely as possible: What is the stuff that makes up who you are, this thing you call "me"? Beyond your name, title, gender, and roles, who are you? Are you a body? Are you a mind? Both? Neither? Are you made up of something more than a body and a mind? I don't know about you, but when I first heard this question, I thought it was ridiculous. *Who am I? Obviously, I am my name, Rajshree. I'm a lawyer, an Indian American, a woman, and I suppose that I'm also my body, along with what I think, feel, and believe.* That was "me." At that time, I'm not even sure I knew what the word *mind* was referring to, exactly, although I used it all the time. My brain was my mind, right? Soon after I began my study of the mind through the lens of the Vedic tradition, I arrived at a very different answer. It doesn't matter if you don't have clear answers to these questions right now. I just want you to start thinking about the different elements that come together to create this system that you call *you*.

If you break it down, you will find that you operate on multiple levels. There's the part that I could then easily recognize, this physical organism called the body. Then there's this nonmaterial, thinking substance called the mind, which I was familiar with, even if I couldn't begin to explain to you what it really was. Then there is this other nonmaterial essence that some people call "spirit" or "soul." I had certainly been exposed to these words since I was a kid, and in some casual way I believed in the soul, but never could I imagine identifying myself with it. Today, I understand this essence as the "heart-mind" or the "Big Mind," but we're not going to get into that just yet.

The Seven Layers of Your Life

When the rishis underwent a scientific observation of their own existence, they saw that there were seven distinct but interconnected layers, or faculties, that make up the whole of who we are. Collectively, this human system is made up of:

- **Body:** The physical matter of cells, organs, bones, and tissues that comprises our anatomy.

- **Breath:** The air that moves in and out of the body, bringing and sustaining life.

- **Mind:** The faculty of perception, including the five senses.

- **Intellect:** The faculty of labeling, judging, categorizing, reasoning, analyzing, and strategizing.

- **Memory:** The faculty that stores all information and our lifetime of experiences.

- **Ego:** The faculty of identity, your personality or sense of "I."

- **Consciousness:** The faculty of pure awareness, also known as "spirit" or "Big Mind."

The rishis didn't view the mind as a single unified entity. Instead, they understood it as a grouping of several distinct faculties. In the Vedic system, "mind" is broken up into three layers: perception, intellect, and memory. Then, existing on another level separate from the body-mind complex is our personal identity—the ego. And of course, on another level separate from it all, there is consciousness, that deeper essence that you might call "spirit." Together, these seven layers form one complete unit. Think of it like a car: you've got the engine, the wheels, the fuel, the steering wheel. They're all doing separate things, but they have to work together to make the car run. Without any one of these parts, the car is incomplete, and it won't function. Each part serves a specific purpose and operates with its own rules.

On one level, each of these faculties functions independently. On another, they're all connected in an intricate system. At any given moment in time, your body is doing one thing, your breath is doing another, and the mind is off doing something else entirely. And yet the workings of each layer are always impacting the others. Fearful or anxious activity in the mind creates a state of high alert in the nervous system, which affects the speed of the breath, which impacts the state of the immune, hormonal, and digestive systems. The reverse is also true—that a dysfunction in your digestive system impacts your nervous system, which negatively affects the breath and all layers of the mind. When your body is sick or tired, you've experienced how it affects your mind, your mood, and your general disposition. It's all connected.

These seven faculties are like different departments of an organization. Each faculty taps into the same innate life force for the battery power to sustain its activity, but they all operate according to their own unique rules for what enhances versus drains energy. You can think of these rules as principles for optimum performance. When the rules are violated, you drain your own well-being, your capabilities, and your personal power.

Body Rules Vs. Mind Rules

The rules aren't the same across the system, and what's good for one faculty isn't necessarily what's best for another. Take the body, for instance. Efficiency and high performance in the body come from *effort and activity*. That's the body's rule for optimum functioning. Body thrives on motion, doing, and acting. Your system is meant to be physically dynamic. That's why you exercise. When the body is highly active, you find yourself with an abundance of energy. On the other hand, being motionless, sitting on the couch all day, will drain your energy, not just physically but mentally. A sedentary lifestyle will not only hurt your health but shorten your life-span, because it takes away your energy. Haven't you seen those headlines that say things like "Sitting All Day Will Kill You, According to Science"? It's true! Inactivity saps the body of its vitality. This is why you go to the gym! You might sit at a desk for hours on end every day, and then you have to get on a treadmill, staring at a parking lot, going nowhere in order to make up for all the inactivity.

Haven't you seen those headlines that say things like "Sitting All Day Will Kill You, According to Science"? It's true!

The mind operates optimally based on the opposite principle. For the mental faculties (lumping together perception, intellect, and memory), you don't need *doing. Mentally,* you don't thrive on work or effort. Mind needs relaxation, stillness, and effortlessness in order to function at its peak. What that means is that the more *activity* in the mind—the more time spent engaged in thinking, worrying, planning, and strategizing—the less sharp, focused, and clear your intellect and perception becomes. When your mind is in overdrive, full of chatter, performance decreases. Your mental faculties stop functioning optimally, and you become more foggy and forgetful. This is when you start losing your car keys, forgetting your appointments, getting stuck in creative blocks, and feeling uncertain in your decision-making. A mind working in overdrive and overtime is the definition of stress, and as research has shown, when stress becomes chronic, it completely erodes your memory faculty.[1]

What happens so often is that you're trying to get the mind to function by the rules of the body, and it just doesn't work very well. Unlike the body, which thrives on activity, the mind operates on the principle of *letting go.* Less effort. Less activity. Effortlessness is the key to a healthy mind! Mind thrives on less trying and less holding on. Let go of the shit that happened yesterday, let go of the shit you're worried will happen tomorrow, let go of what your boyfriend or girlfriend said, let go of the job you didn't get or the client that dropped you. Let go of all this mental debris, and suddenly, without even trying, there it is: a mind functioning at peak performance, totally in the present moment. A mind that is overflowing with energy, clarity, and creativity. If you can let go, your mind can thrive more. But the irony is that the more you actively *try* to let go, the more the shit sticks. The thing is, you don't have to try. Letting go happens naturally as a result of increasing your innate life force. The more energy in your system, the more the mind moves toward where it naturally wants to go: a place of effortlessness and energy efficiency.

For 99 percent of people, the faculty that's exhausted and draining the entire system is the mind, not the body. The mind is the biggest energy hog you can imagine! The overwhelming majority of your life force goes toward sustaining just those three mental faculties and their endless activity and effort. Effort on the mind level is what's draining you more than anything else, but you've never learned how to address it. Instead, self-help and positive thinking techniques teach you to add even more effort on top of all the mental activity that's already sapping you dry.

The problem is that we've never been taught that the mind operates on completely different principles than the body does. So we keep trying to apply the same principle to the mind as we do to the body (more activity, more effort, more doing), and it's not working so well. There are so many people who are doing "everything right" for their health and well-being, but they're still not functioning anywhere close to their potential. They're taking vitamins and supplements, they're eating clean, they're going to spin class and sleeping eight hours, but their minds are still exhausted and ineffective. Why? It's because vitamins and vegetables and exercise fuel the body, but they're not doing anything to address the mental overactivity that's draining the lion's share of the batteries that are meant to power your entire system. It's the unnecessary chatter in the mind, the negative emotions, the limiting beliefs that are sapping life force and draining the whole system—and the reality is that all the green juice and protein shakes and workout classes in the world are just not enough to address that.

If your energy is lagging and your life is lukewarm despite all your best efforts to energize yourself, it's a sign that you need to be looking at your mind. It's time to recognize two big secrets: (1) Your mind is the biggest energy hog of the entire system. (2) When you're dealing with the mind, you have to play by the mind's rules—meaning operating from *effortlessness* rather than effort.

Your Mental Machinery

Your mind operates on three different levels. Think of it like an iceberg: there's the tip of the iceberg, the waterline, and the enormous base that's submerged underwater, hidden from sight. When you look at an iceberg, you can only see that very top portion that sticks up above the surface of the water. You have no idea that 90 percent of the iceberg's mass lies below the surface of the ocean, invisible to the eye. The iceberg is a classic analogy for the mind, used by Freud and others, because the two share a similar structure. The tip of the iceberg can be compared to the *conscious mind*—the tiny sliver of thought and perception that we are actually aware of in our day-to-day lives. Moving down a level, there's the *preconscious mind* that hovers right around and just below the waterline, which consists of all the things you're not currently thinking about but could easily bring to mind if prompted. If I asked you to recall what you had for dinner last night or where you went to elementary school, your mind would immediately dip into the preconscious mind to grab an answer. Another level below, you'll find the submerged portion of the iceberg: the *unconscious mind*, and a lifetime's worth of stored experiences, beliefs, perceptions, feelings, and memories that you may or may not be aware of or have access to. Then, if you go all the way down to the bottom of the iceberg, you reach the ocean itself, which is your faculty of *consciousness*—the Big Mind.

Let's start at the tip of the iceberg, where we find the faculties of perception and intellect, or what in Vedanta is called *manas* and *buddhi*. The Vedic tradition describes this part of the mind as being the closest to the external world that we take in through our five senses. It's also the furthest from the innermost, true Self. While perception moves across all layers of the iceberg, the intellect (not to be confused with the Intelligence that is synonymous with consciousness) moves only around the tip. For now, we're going to focus on the intellect, the part of our mental hardware that uses up the most of our internal batteries.

Intellect: The Control Center

The intellect is a powerful faculty that can either serve us or give us lots of trouble. It's where all surface-level thought, planning, decision-making, analyzing, judging, labeling, and strategizing takes place—in short, it's our "thinking brain." We use the intellect to process information from the environment that comes in via our senses. This task-oriented, "figure shit out" faculty is what helps us make sense of the world and navigate our way through every situation in life. Anything we do with the data we currently have access to, whether above or below the waterline of awareness, is the work of the intellect. Physiologically, the seat of the intellect is the frontal cortex of the brain, the neurological "control center" that sits right behind the forehead. This part of the mind doesn't innovate or create new ideas or possibilities. It accounts for maybe 10 percent of our total capacity, but it consumes more of our time and energy than any other faculty.

Memory: The Data Storage Center

From the tip of the iceberg we move down to the water level, the place from which we can quickly access information that's only partially submerged. This is the *preconscious* mind, and it's where we first encounter the faculty of memory (*chitta*). Information from the preconscious mind isn't in your frontal cortex right at this moment, you're not thinking about it or analyzing it, but if I remind you, you could access it almost immediately.

There is a constant exchange between the conscious and the preconscious mind, a sort of data-sharing partnership where information is constantly being called up to the surface to be processed by the intellect, and then filed away in the memory bank until it's needed again in the future. The information may appear different when it comes back up again at a later moment in time, but often we are just calling up the same old thoughts, ideas, and perceptions over and over again.

Chitta: The Submerged Mind

Below these two levels of awareness, there's a tremendous amount of activity also going on in the submerged mind. The vast and powerful base of the iceberg is home to the deeper portions of the memory faculty—your mental data storage center. The memory bank holds a massive amount of data, collected over your entire lifetime, which can travel back and forth from the tip of the iceberg down to its depths. In neurological terms, the memory bank corresponds with the *limbic brain*, the emotion and memory-formation center located at the back of the head near the base of the skull. In Vedic tradition, we call it *chitta*, which refers to the "subconscious": the vast storehouse of past experiences that dictates the way we react to things in the present. It's what creates our perceptions of life and our immediate, knee-jerk emotional reactions to everything we experience.

The memory bank holds a massive amount of data, collected over your entire lifetime, which can travel back and forth from the tip of the iceberg down to its depths.

Chitta holds the record of everything you've ever experienced. It's chock-full of impressions from throughout your lifetime— some of it stored there knowingly and some of it processed and filed away without any awareness on your part. You don't need to be conscious of what's happening in order for it to do its job. Experiences, perceptions, information, emotions, and desires— all of this gets stored beneath the waterline, with the more recent and relevant material sitting closer to the surface. Deep down in the submerged part of the iceberg, we also find everything that we've suppressed or blocked from our conscious awareness— unpleasant thoughts, difficult emotions, painful memories, and the parts of ourselves that we have a hard time accepting. You can push these down below the surface of the water, but they go on existing in the depths of the memory bank.

Brain Drain

If you look at the entire iceberg, it's obvious that the most powerful part is the base. That's what determines the shape of the whole iceberg and dictates the direction in which it will drift. But where do we spend all of our time? Not down here in the powerful base layer. We're skimming above the surface of the water, operating out of our frontal cortex. So much of our life is spent in frontal cortex activities of thinking, processing, reasoning, planning, decision-making, worrying, and judging. It almost never stops. The intellect is constantly processing the information we have access to in the moment, whether we need that information or not.

We use this part of the mind more than any other, but it's obvious if you look at the whole iceberg that the frontal cortex is really the smallest aspect of the iceberg from which we function. It's only the surface layer of the mind. When we restrict ourselves to the surface, we block off access to our deeper potentiality, such as insight, intuition, and creativity. This part of the mind and its incessant activity is draining a *significant* amount of battery power and potential. You know when you click the battery icon on your computer and it tells you which application is "using significant energy"? That energy hog would be the intellect.

I'm not saying the intellect is good or bad. It's neither. The problem is that we use it far more than necessary and we don't know how to turn it off. Think of your intellect as being like one of many rooms in a large house. What if you confined yourself to only one room to use for all the things you need to do? It's certainly possible to do that; it's just not a very smart or efficient way of doing things. When you limit yourself to one room, you're ignoring all of the other possibilities that can arise from using the other rooms of the house.

The activity of the intellect consumes a tremendous amount of vital force. I don't know if you've ever noticed this, but in my observation of thousands of people, I've seen that those who are the most intellectual are often the least lively and spontaneous. Their vital force is usually the lowest in the room. They are so filled with thoughts, information, and concepts that they're missing the joy of experience. They spend most of their energy analyzing every little thing in their lives, and it's burning out the battery. Recently the medical profession labeled a new disease that can now be billed to insurance companies. It's called "burnout syndrome." Funnily enough, medical professionals, whose work requires them to rely heavily on their intellects, suffer from it more than any other profession—but lawyers are a close second! Just ask yourself: How many people do you know who are highly intellectual but also vibrant, joyful, and expressive? These kinds of people exist, but they're rare.

The True Cost of Thinking

The intellect, with its incessant thinking, uses up far more energy than we realize. From the moment we wake up to the moment we fall asleep at night (and sometimes during sleep too), the intellect is generating an endless stream of repetitive thoughts and judgments. The energy cost of this nonstop activity is huge. Look at your own mind: while you're doing everything you do, you're also thinking. While you're making coffee, talking to a friend, driving to work, running errands, exercising, taking care of your kids, or watching TV, there are simultaneously thousands of thoughts running: interpreting, judging, commenting, mind-wandering, self-talk. And guess what? Ninety-five percent of the time, your mind is talking about things that don't matter. It's using up your precious life force for no reason.

The reality of our hyperconnected, always-busy modern lives is that the intellect almost never shuts down—not even when you're sleeping. It's still using (and draining) energy. Your head is still running through every little worry and concern: how your day was, the conversation with your mother-in-law, planning your upcoming vacation. The frontal cortex is still online all night—it's a little quieter, but it's still processing huge volumes of information. You know that feeling when you're kind of half-asleep, but you're not entirely sure if you're sleeping? A part of your brain is asleep, but the intellect in still in full swing. You feel like you've been thinking all night, and that's because you have. You wake up exhausted—in a way, more exhausted than when you went to sleep. That's because you left the computer running all night long. The frontal cortex was still going! The computer is still using energy to run and process files all night, so it doesn't charge fully. You don't quite get to 100 percent battery. Your intellect was thinking and worrying, and your limbic brain was cycling through the storehouse of memories in your sleep and dreams all night. Sometimes a memory of something that happened during the day or earlier is triggered, but you didn't sleep deeply enough to process it and let it go. Is it any wonder you feel as though you woke up on the wrong side of the bed and walk around feeling "off" all day?

We know that thoughts are nothing more than electrical impulses of intelligence. Scientists can measure thoughts in electromagnetic signals as they arise, and according to cardiologist and author Deepak Chopra, we have somewhere between 60,000 and 80,000 in a day. Do you think any of us have 60,000 original thoughts on any given Wednesday? Nope! We're lucky if we have six original thoughts in a day. The rest of our thoughts are redundant and unproductive. We're telling ourselves the same old story again and again—different day, different triggers, same frustrations and anxieties. All this thinking is like having too many open files on a computer, which drains the battery and slows down the whole device. Imagine if you could just reduce that 60,000 thoughts to 50,000 thoughts. You'd already be so much more vibrant! You'd have a glow in your complexion and an extra spring in your step. People would start asking you what you've been doing differently, if you've lost weight or been doing yoga. You'd be so much more alive, connected, dynamic, and creative. You'd also be saving yourself a lot of energy—energy that could be put toward more meaningful and life-enhancing pursuits.

When you're mentally exhausted, your response to whatever's happening in your life (even if it's a good thing!) becomes I can't handle this. It's too much. I'm overwhelmed. I feel out of control.

The lower the number of thoughts in your mind, the more present, aware, decisive, focused, perceptive, clear, strategic, creative, and innovative your mind will be. The less mental activity, the more optimized the function of every mental faculty. There is a direct link between the amount of energy in your mental faculties, the number of thoughts you have, and the function of the mind. Lower energy means more thoughts and lower function. Higher energy means better function and fewer thoughts. I hope you're catching on to the fact that the simplest way to become more mindful, more focused, more clear, and more creative is to charge up your mind with the power of life energy.

Stress: The Mind in Survival Mode

In Western cultures, we've been fooled into thinking that thinking is good for us. Thinking has its value, but thinking the same thing over and over again—often for 5, 10, or God knows how many more years—is clearly inefficient. To function in life, we need to plan, think, figure, judge, and interpret. But to go on doing it over and over again in the same ways is a waste of time, effort, and energy . . . and ultimately a waste of life itself. As a lawyer, I would often get fixated on a case. The same case ran through my mind morning, noon, and night, often long after it was over. Looking back at it now seems crazy. I had so many cases to attend to, and I was running on empty, but at the level of intellect, I was revving the engine over and over again and going nowhere. I was stressed out all the time. I started losing my focus and efficiency, which only created more thoughts of self-judgment and worry. My mind was in overdrive.

This is a state that's all too familiar to most people. Too many open files in the mind is what we call "stress" in the broadest sense of the word. Stress is fundamentally a by-product of low vital force on a mental level, and it's an energetically costly state that wears down the whole system over time. When the mind is overworked and overtired, thoughts, perceptions, and outlook become weaker, our reactions to life's events become negative, and the whole system goes into "defense mode," directing huge amounts of inner resources to protecting itself from perceived threats to its survival. When you're mentally exhausted, your response to whatever's happening in your life (even if it's a good thing!) becomes *I can't handle this. It's too much. I'm overwhelmed. I feel out of control.*

Here's a simple definition of stress, from the perspective of energy: stress is when your demand exceeds your capacity. Too much demand, not enough capacity (meaning time and energy) to meet the demand. You have so many things to do and not enough time and energy to do it all. You have to ask yourself, then, what's draining all of your time and energy? There are some external things that you probably have little control over, and then there's the endless mental activity that's sapping your efficiency, productivity, clarity, and vitality.

Generally speaking, each one of us is born with a fully charged battery of life force, and we all have 24 hours in a day to get things done. Assuming, we all have the same amount of internal resources available to us, and yet some build empires and move mountains while others struggle to keep on top of the basic daily demands of life. Why? If one person is mentally exhausted and low in vital force while the other has high mental energy, the latter will find themselves able, willing, and ready to deal with much more in life—with a smile on their face!

When you have less mental energy, you also have less efficiency—which translates into less time to do the things you need or want to do. As a result, even the smallest things are experienced as a demand that feels "too much." There's not enough energy, not enough time, and not enough space in the mind to tackle daily life, so you experience life as "stressful"—even if the "stressor" is something joyful, like a wedding or an exciting new business opportunity. If you want to address your stress, trying to remove the external demands from your life is not the best solution. The reality is that it may not be possible for you to shorten your to-do list. To me, having only enough energy to get through what has to be done is not much of a life. What about the enthusiasm, excitement, and energy for the things you really want to do? This is the difference between existing and living. The way to do this is to conserve and supercharge your mental energy, blowing out the intellect's extra chatter of doubts, complaints, judging, and negativity. It can't be said enough: more energy means higher levels of cognitive function and higher levels of happiness.

Optimize Your Intellect

Remember the effortlessness principle of the mind: if you want your mind to function optimally, reducing unnecessary mental activity is the key.

What any good parent or friend will say to someone who's obsessing over a problem is "Just sleep on it" or "Step away from it for a few hours." We say this because we need to shut down the frontal cortex, and when the frontal cortex quiets down, we are able to tap into the state of flow, mental clarity, creativity, and insight. New information becomes available when we quiet down. Suddenly we figure out the best course of action.

We suddenly come up with a new idea or a new logo, or we remember where we left our keys. For this moment of "eureka" to arise requires energy and mental space. Dropping thinking, even for just a moment, conserves energy and gives the mind a moment to settle into a deeper layer of awareness so that a new outlook can arise.

Have you noticed that when you're in an unexpected situation or new setting, you can think on your feet more easily than when you're stuck in the same old rut? It's because you are forced to innovate, forced to transcend the intellect, in a new situation. You can't just default to repetitive thinking. When I'm speaking in front of large groups, I don't have the luxury of time to mull things over. My lectures are often Q&A sessions with an audience, where they're asking questions about their lives and what matters the most to them. It's kind of like improv. There are 500 people with unique personal challenges in the room, all asking for my attention. When someone asks a question, I'm forced to just be in the moment. My judging, analyzing intellect shuts down and my responses are spontaneous. That's what happens in a flow state. We move beyond same-old thinking and into the present moment.

This temporary shutting down of the intellect during a moment of flow can actually be observed on a neurological level. When you're in that flow state—completely present and blissfully absorbed in what you're doing, caught up in that elusive, losing-all-sense-of-time state of creativity and peak performance—something happens in that brain called *transient hypofrontality*.[2] What that literally means is that your frontal cortex temporarily slows down or deactivates. When that happens, you dip into the enormous, submerged base of the iceberg, and moments of clarity, intuition, and deep insight bubble up from the depths of the ocean. When the intellect finally calms down, you're able to tap into all the other parts of the mind that were being overshadowed by the tyranny of the thinking mind. Supercharge your mind with life force, and you naturally and effortlessly dip into that state of flow.

In Your Mind, What's Old Is New

It's not just the endless thinking of the intellect that consumes energy and slows down the system. Beneath the surface of the water, there are hundreds of programs that we're not even aware of, running and consuming energy all the time.

If we want new ideas, new choices, and different actions—if we want to venture outside the box of our limiting beliefs—then we need to delete the stored cookies or at least shut down the open tabs.

The direction of our thoughts, and the movement of the whole iceberg, is driven by the submerged base of the iceberg. That's where most of the data is stored. It's the mind's hard drive. Most computers keep a "history" that predicts what you're going to search for based on your prior searches. This more or less sums up your life. There aren't a lot of new things happening! We are operating from our past events, spinning in the same circle. This is where our limiting beliefs are born: from the storehouse of past memories, many of them going back to early childhood, that lead us to draw certain conclusions about who we are and how the world works. If we want new ideas, new choices, and different actions—if we want to venture outside the box of our limiting beliefs—then we need to delete the stored cookies or at least shut down the open tabs.

The overwhelming majority of your thoughts are driven by old emotional patterns, experiences, and beliefs you formed in childhood. This is what we've been calling the "conditioned mind." It's like a bad sitcom that you watch again and again and again. The old rerun is funny once or twice, but then, the third time you watch the episode, it's just a way to keep yourself busy, and the fourth or fifth time, you feel bored and frustrated and exhausted from it. The same thing is going on within your own mind, in your thoughts. You're also getting fed up with the same old thinking and the same old emotions. Internally you are doing the same things, getting the same results, getting frustrated, and living a lukewarm life. The only thing that's different is the external object of your focus and attention. One of the biggest things to realize is that the frontal cortex is almost all repetitive thinking, ideas, and beliefs. It doesn't really yield any great results. You keep doing the same thing again and again, like Pavlov's dog or a rat in a maze.

What you hold on to in your memory and send back and forth to the intellect creates a huge drain in life force. Files in the limbic brain, including unresolved, partially processed thoughts, emotions, and memories, are using energy by staying open. If I remind you of a negative file—an ex who broke your heart, a business deal that went sour, or a friend who betrayed you—how quickly you feel the emotion associated with it tells you how powerful it is and how much energy it's draining. Even if you don't know how to delete the file from the hard drive, you should at least learn how to close out the tab. These open files are what drain the life out of you and potentially slow down your whole system. Again, your mind's operating system holds an almost unimaginable amount of data, but it can't hold everything. There may be an infinite amount of storage space, but you may not have the capacity to hold it without crashing or slowing down.

If there are a hundred files open on the computer, even if you don't see those files, they are drawing on the battery. They're consuming your mental capacity, your talents, your energy, your intelligence, your wisdom, and your intuition. They're impacting everything.

It takes energy to keep things occupying the internal space that you don't need, that you're not conscious of—beliefs and assumptions that worked for you 10 years ago but that don't make any sense in your life today. Maybe it's the belief that nobody is there for you that was created when you were a toddler and your mother was barely around, or the assumption based on a past trauma that the world is not a safe place and you have to constantly defend yourself against potential threats. Returning to the beginner's mind, the free and spontaneous mind you had as a child, is what is needed for optimum mental functioning. The more you operate from beginner's mind, the more effortless you are, and the more you can let go of what doesn't serve you. But instead of letting go, you waste all of your energy trying to hold on and keeping everything in its place.

The things you're holding on to occupy space and use up energy. If you keep downloading apps on your phone until the storage is almost used up, the phone eventually stops working as well. If you have too many things downloaded, whether they're useful apps or not-so-useful ones that you never open, it slows down the hard drive. When I get a new phone, the first thing I do is get rid of the apps that I don't want. I know that if I have too many apps running, my phone's battery will burn out more quickly, and I'll have to charge it more often. Internally, having too many programs clutters our mental landscape. You have to recharge your battery every day. Enhancing your innate life force is the quickest way to recharge the entire mind *and* delete old files from the hard drive so that the computer, and all of its hardware and software, functions better.

EXERCISE: What Programs Are Running in Your System?

I'd like to do a quick exercise to support you in identifying some of the most energy-depleting programs that are running in your mind. I want you to really see how your mind is unnecessarily using up your inner resources, abilities, and energy. In addition, this exercise will become valuable in the next chapter to get you in touch with what you're holding on to in the deeper layers of mind and emotion.

As you can see, page 73 is blank, and it's been divided into four columns. Please grab a pen and give yourself 5 to 10 minutes to go through this exercise. In the first column, write down a list of 10 things that have recently been on your mind. We're talking about things in your life that are taking your attention and energy . . . your product launch, your boss, colleagues, finances, children, parents, climate change—you name it. Whatever it is, just write down a single word or phrase to represent it. If you are contemplating a career change, write "career change." You don't have to include details on what, where, when, or how. And if you're having trouble identifying what's been on your mind, try looking at what you talk about with friends and family. What we talk about the most is usually a pretty good indication of what's going on internally. Here's an example of what your list might look like:

1. Career change

2. Paying off debt

3. Recent weight gain

4. Conflict with spouse or significant other

5. Worries about political situation

6. Recurring health complaint

7. New diet

8. Taking care of aging mother

9. Car purchase

10. Saving to go back to school

In the second column, next to each item, indicate the emotion that's generated by the thought of that situation, using a "+" for positive emotion or "-" for negative emotion. Sometimes you might find that a situation—particularly something big like a career change—creates both positive and negative emotions, in which case you can put both a + and a - sign.

When you're finished, add up all the positives and negatives. What do your results look like? Is your list 10 percent, 50 percent, 90 percent positive or negative? Over nearly three decades of working with and observing thousands of people, what I have discovered is that, on average, the main contents of most people's minds are around 80 percent negative. I ask you: How does your mind compare?

We'll come back to this exercise in the next chapter to explore it more deeply (and that's when you'll fill in the remaining columns). For now, suffice it to say that positive thoughts generate positive emotions, and negative thoughts generate negative emotions. Obviously, negative thoughts and emotions drain our life and energy, while positive thoughts and emotions uplift energy and enhance our quality of life. If we want to enhance our energy and create the space for more positive emotions to naturally arise, we need to address the negativity that the mind gets stuck in.

List 10 Things	Positive (+) or Negative (-)	Emotion Generated	Past, Now, Future

CHAPTER 5

The Past Is Present

There's a great movie you may have seen called *Groundhog Day* about a TV weatherman (played by Bill Murray) who wakes up one morning horrified to find that he is reliving the previous day all over again: same events, experiences, and people, down to the tiniest detail. Murray's character finds himself living this strange Twilight Zone day after day, stuck in an eternal yesterday.

The movie (which was actually directed by a Buddhist filmmaker) offers a good look at how the mind works from a Vedic perspective. The rishis saw that one of the mind's basic tendencies is to get stuck in the past. But unlike in the movie, in real life, you have no idea that your mind is reliving the past over and over again. Things around you look different, so you think they've changed. But internally, you're still just replaying the same old tape of the conditioned mind. This is what the mind does: it brings the past into the present, then it takes the present, which is based on the past, and it uses that to create what looks like the future—but really is just another re-creation of the past! That's right: your future is nothing more than the reappearance of your past in a "new" form!

We're not fully aware of it, but we spend our lives repeating the same experiences and often the same mistakes. The mind gets stuck in something that happened in that past that it can't let go of, which generates more or less the same type of thoughts, which then produce similar actions, which lead to the same or similar results. Our results might look different because the situation, the person, or the object of focus has changed, but make no mistake, we are still running in the same circle. Remember the saying "Insanity is doing the same thing and expecting different results"? Welcome to Groundhog Day!

If we want to bring the mind back into the present moment, into a state of flow, connected to the source of energy and intelligence within, we have to first become aware of where it's stuck, which is in the past and in the future. When we're in the present moment, the mind is still, calm, powerful, and focused. There's not unnecessary activity. The mental activity that takes us out of the moment is related to one of two things: the past or the future. If you look at your own mind, you'll notice that you're constantly caught up in thoughts of the past and future—and in the negative emotions that are generated by those thoughts. This is the vicious mental cycle that's sapping our mental vitality and creating stress throughout the system.

If we want to bring the mind back into the present moment, into a state of flow, connected to the source of energy and intelligence within, we have to first become aware of where it's stuck.

Have you ever wondered where thoughts come from? They pop into our heads all day long without warning, and many of them we don't even want. So what the hell?! Where on earth are they coming from? According to Vedanta, the root of all thought is the past (*smriti*). Every thought, positive or negative, is created by the past. We like to think we're responding to life in the moment with a fresh mind, but the reality is very different. We learned in the last chapter that the thoughts that we're aware of at the tip of the iceberg are coming from the memory bank in the part that's submerged. We see something in the environment, which stimulates our faculty of perception (either consciously or unconsciously), which triggers a thought to bubble up to the surface from the deep, submerged expanses of the memory bank. To me, this is a pretty scary idea. Are we really just doomed to relive the same shit again and again? On some level, yes.

When you see a pit bull on the street, you're not just seeing a pit bull—you might be seeing the pit bull that attacked you when you were a kid, or you might see the sweet, loving pit bull that your friend recently rescued. The same thing happens with stimuli in your internal landscape. Let's say you just got engaged, and you've been imagining what your future marriage might look like. Your thoughts about your marriage aren't just a pure, in-the-moment response to the idea of being married. They're being influenced by all the data your mind has gathered, stored, and tagged "marriage," "divorce," "family," and the rest of the related list, which is endless. It's observations of your parents' interactions when you were a child, movies you've seen that explore themes of marriage and divorce, Instagram photos of your married friends looking happy, and conversations with friends about their struggles with their spouses. You might think you're just imagining your married future, but below the level of awareness, your mind is taking a journey through the past.

Once a thought bubbles up to the surface, the intellect judges, analyzes, and dissects that thought. It observes the thought from every angle and chops it up into a million little pieces. Even if we're experiencing or learning something for the first time, the mind is still digging up old files to influence the way we perceive it. This is what we call our *conditioning*, and it's why the same things happen to us over and over again. It's also a big part of why it's so difficult to break out of old patterns. If we want something new in our lives, we need to be aware of what we're holding on to in our memory bank so that we can make a conscious choice about whether to use or discard that information. That's something we've never been taught how to do. It is possible to clear out the files that are cluttering the memory bank, and we'll learn techniques for doing that later in the book. But the crucial first step is to become aware of how much the past is robbing us in the present—and the future.

Who we are, how we live right now, AND how we create our future is being decided by the past. And I don't think you need me to tell you that it's not just the joyful memories and good times that are shaping our outlook.

The Vedic understanding of mind says that *chitta*, memory, is what defines our personality and determines the way we see the world. Growing up in India, for instance, I was hardwired with communal thinking. On the plus side, I naturally gravitate toward collaboration and group activities. On the down side, my knee-jerk reaction is to always think about what's best for the group, often discounting my own needs and desires.

The past is driving the direction of our thoughts, which dictates how we act, which in turn determines what we create in our life, which further cements the beliefs and outlooks we've created based on past experiences. That means that who we are, how we live right now, AND how we create our future is being decided by the past. And I don't think you need me to tell you that it's not just the joyful memories and good times that are shaping our outlook. The biggest part of what's driving us and generating the struggles we keep repeating over and over again is the *negative past*. It's this endless cycle of past-generated negative thoughts and emotions that drains more mental energy than anything else imaginable. Not only do we suffer the injury of whatever happened in the past that we didn't like or thought was unfair, but now we suffer again and drain ourselves even more because we're still carrying it with us into the present and the potential future. The past event is tainting *this moment*, the moment from which we create our future.

And what about the future? As much as your mind is stuck in the past, it can also be stuck in the future. If you could flip through the archives of your memory bank, you'd find that what's stored there are not only memories of things that have already happened but also memories of your worries, dreams, and desires for the future . . . which are entirely based on your past experiences. On the level of the mind, *the future is nothing more than the anticipated past.* We take the bits of information we've gathered—the learning, experiences, data, ideas, assumptions, ideologies, and belief systems collected over the years—and we project them onto a present that has not yet arrived. This journey of past and future—dwelling on something that happened and then worrying about something that might happen—is one of the mind's most energy-inefficient programs. Why? Because it never stops running!

Take a moment to sincerely look at yourself. How much of your time and energy is spent thinking about what happened to you yesterday or five years ago? What about what might happen tomorrow or in six months? You know that you can't change your past, and the future may or may not end up how you imagine it, but have you ever stopped to consider how much time is being wasted on this? If you're being honest, the answer is going to be *a lot.* This constant oscillation between the past and the future is simply the nature of your mind. For most people, as we've seen, at least 80 percent of this past and future thinking is negative. If 8 out of 10 files that are running in your mind are negative, this is naturally going to color your perception and outlook of what's happening right now. You won't see things clearly; you'll see them through the filter of that negativity: *This always happens to me, This is never a good idea, I don't know if I can do it, I'm just not sure,* and on and on.

Look at your own life: If 10 positive things happen to you and one negative thing happens, what do you remember? Someone gives you 10 compliments and one insult. What has more energy, the insult or the compliments? You have 10 amazing things happen throughout the course of your workday—you meet a new friend for lunch, you have a good talk with your boss, your tasks go smoothly—but you get stuck in traffic for an extra 30 minutes on your way home, and you're late for a dinner party. Which do you focus on more? What takes up more of your time—the positivity or the negativity? For most of us, it's the negativity. Again, this is just the nature of the mind. Freud said that all stored memories have a particular energetic charge to them, and the charge of negative memories is much stronger than the charge of positive or neutral memories. Modern science, too, tells us that our brain is hardwired with a negative bias that's so automatic that it can be detected at the earliest stage of information processing. We are simply built with a greater sensitivity to unpleasant news. Of course this is valuable in that it can keep us out of harm's way. However, it means the same bad news bias is also at work in every aspect of our lives.

To say that negativity has a greater electrical charge means that it consumes more energy. That's true whether we are actively remembering the difficult things that have happened to us or trying to suppress them. It takes a LOT of energy to keep painful or traumatic memories submerged below the waterline, where we can't see them. The greater the negative charge, the more often the memory gets triggered, and the more energy is required to sweep it under the rug.

Of course, reflecting on the past isn't always a bad thing. We can look to the past for lessons to help us understand our present and improve our future. But let's be honest: that's not really what we're doing most of the time. We're thinking about the past because we're stuck in something we can't let go of. A few years ago, a friend of mine was driving her car and got into an accident on the 405 freeway. Ever since then, driving for her is always associated with thoughts of *It's too much, It's unsafe, I'm not good at this, I don't like this.* She might try to block those thoughts from her awareness, but they're always there. Her mind is still stuck in the accident, and it affects her feelings about driving (and herself as a driver) right now, which she carries into her future. Instead of learning the lesson of what she did wrong that led to the accident, she allows the experience to generate regret, anxiety, and judgment toward herself and the act of driving. This is what we do: the lesson is so simple, but we create a huge story around it, and we get stuck in that story. She can't go back and undo that accident, and yet her mind will not let it go. There's not a thing in the world that we can do about the past, but it's still affecting our entire life: our work, relationships, health, well-being, and enjoyment of life. In my friend's case, it's not difficult to see how this cycle is draining her mental vitality and vibrancy every time it gets triggered. It's creating more mental effort, more thought, and more negative charge every time she gets in the car.

We like to think that we're "figuring things out" by worrying about them. But tell me, when has worrying ever helped you find a solution?

Getting stuck in the future can be equally draining. Thoughts of the future can bring excitement and hope, but more often they bring fear, worry, anxiety, and, at the extreme end, panic. This robs us of the present moment too! So much of what happens in life is beyond our control, and things may or may not turn out the way we plan. Even if the future we fear does arrive, operating in the present from a place of worry doesn't help us in the now.

We like to think that we're "figuring things out" by worrying about them. But tell me, when has worrying ever helped you find a solution? If you're worried about the possibility of losing your job, you are now unable to focus or perform well at work. If you're stressing about your financial situation so much that you can't sleep at night, that takes away the creative energy you need to develop alternative income streams. Your worry and anxiety are probably affecting your health—that takes even more energy—and they're fogging your thinking and decision-making. Can you see how you're just creating a self-fulfilling prophecy? This is how your future is killing your present.

Emotional Drain

As a general rule, the more time we spend in the past and future, the more we get stuck in re-creating the past and the negative emotions that come with it. The biggest drain is in the emotions and the self-judgments about the emotions that are triggered. Emotions are pure energy. They're simple movement of life force up or down in the system (hence the term *e-motion*). If left to run their course, the emotions will come and go easily. An emotion with a negative charge *consumes* energy, while a positively charged emotion *enhances* energy. When our life force is high, we treat our emotions with less judgment and allow them to come and go like a line in water. When life force is low, however, a negative emotion can create a groove as deep as the Grand Canyon.

Every negative emotion is a response to either the past or the future. It's never in the present moment. Look at anger: it's always about an event, situation, or person that you don't like and refuse to accept. And then there's anxiety, which arises when you're fixating on the possibility of something going wrong in the future. We call these emotions negative not because they're innately bad or wrong but because they create disturbances in the mind that negatively affect your energy, your outlook, and your quality of life. Think about what happens to you when you're pissed off or sad. Do you have more energy and focus, or are you distracted and on edge? What about when you feel joy or love—how does that impact your energy and focus? A positive emotion is called positive because it increases and replenishes life force. It brings you back into the present moment. When you're filled with gratitude for a loved one or when you receive good news, notice that you walk around the rest of the day with more buoyancy, excitement, and energy.

The rishis realized that everything we want in life is directly related to our ability to let go of the past and the future and return to the present moment. That's the whole spiritual path, the entire purpose of yoga and meditation and therapy and stress reduction and all these other things we do to improve ourselves. To the degree that the mind is in the present, we experience all these things we want in life: happiness, love, connection, clarity, focus, vitality, a feeling of being fully alive.

When we're not present, positive feelings and moments are fleeting. To go back to the marriage example, getting engaged might be one of the happiest experiences of your life. But it only takes a few hours or a few days for the mind to step in and say, "Man, I hope this lasts." Or you start to worry about paying for the wedding or get stuck in some annoyance at your future spouse. You'll notice that this happens even more quickly when your system is depleted. When energy is low, the mind gets more stuck in the journey of past and future. It brings more negative thoughts and emotions. As a result, the positive experience becomes even more short-lived because you can't be present with it. You wish you could enjoy the moment, but the mind is too caught up somewhere else to enjoy being here.

Emotions of the Past: The Anger Spectrum

When we find ourselves thinking about the past, we might feel nostalgia or love as we reflect on the good times. But is that what your mind lingers on? Probably not. The mind quickly gravitates to the things that didn't work so well. We fixate on the struggles and hardships of the past, which generally brings feelings of anger, regret, guilt, and blame—what I call "the anger spectrum" of emotion. Anger is always related to something that happened that we don't like and can't accept. It begins with impatience, annoyance, and irritation, moving further into agitation and frustration, and eventually on to full-blown anger, hostility, rage, and violence—and that's just Phase 1. It's not the end. So, then what happens?

Let's say you got angry at your husband or kids. After the anger bursts out of you, what often follows is a sense of regret. With that we enter Phase 2. *I know I'm tired, and it's been a long day, but I shouldn't have yelled at my children. I don't want them to grow up hating me.* The regret phase begins with subtle questioning of the moment that's already passed. If, at that moment, you could say, *Oh, well, something happened that made me angry, and I got impatient and yelled at the people I love,* you'd apologize and move on to a new moment. But you don't drop it there. You just keep questioning yourself and regretting your actions: *Why did I do that? I shouldn't have done that. What's wrong with me?*

If you don't stop at the second phase, that questioning grows, leading into Phase 3: guilt. It's no longer just questioning; now there's a sense of self-criticism, belittling yourself, and feeling flawed or inadequate. You start doubting your own worthiness. In the guilt phase, you're using your own energy against yourself to beat yourself up. You start to "eternalize" your behavior: *I always do that. There must be something wrong with me.*

How long can you continue beating yourself up? At some point you run out of energy to keep punching. The body and mind are bruised. You keep telling yourself, *I'm bad, I'm no good, I always mess up,* and you just reabsorb all this self-directed negativity. This brings you to Phase 4: blame. You start needing to justify your actions and do something to alleviate the guilt, so you create stories, explanations, and reasons for why you did what you did. It's a way to try to release the huge weight of the guilt. *I did it because my husband made me angry. I did it because this is what my mom used to do to me when I was a kid. I did it because work has been so stressful lately.* I'm not saying these reasons aren't valid—they may be. But you're really just repeating them to yourself so you can live with the guilt. Most of the time, you start with self-blame. If you've been blaming yourself for something you did wrong, you can only do it for so long before you start pointing the finger to someone or something else. And if you blame someone else long enough, sooner or later the cycle comes back and you start blaming yourself again.

The test to see if you've learned a lesson from the past is this: Are you happy about how you've grown, or are you moaning and complaining about what went wrong?

Here's the worst part of this whole thing: Each time the anger cycle repeats itself, it becomes more intense. You move further along the anger spectrum. Irritation becomes frustration, frustration becomes hostility, and hostility becomes rage. Each time you shift to the right on the spectrum, unless you find a way to rejuvenate and return to center, the angry thoughts and emotions only become stronger and consume more of your energy. The lower your energy, the more you're going to get stuck spinning in this cycle.

It's very possible to get stuck in an anger cycle over a single situation for years and even decades, even though you can't do a thing about the situation itself. You might say you're looking to the past to understand the lesson there, but if you had learned the lesson, you wouldn't be angry and resentful anymore. The moment you learn the lesson, the moment you find meaning in the situation, your energy flips. You feel expanded, excited, and empowered, ready to drop the past and move forward. The anger naturally drops off, and you arrive back in the present moment, ready to live right now. The test to see if you've learned a lesson from the past is this: Are you happy about how you've grown, or are you moaning and complaining about what went wrong?

Guilt: Slowly Sapping Your Life Force

The most drawn-out, energy-crushing stage of the anger cycle is guilt. It's one of the most toxic and draining emotions we can experience. It manipulates and changes our cellular structure, and it's likely that it even alters the expression of our genes. Studies have shown that people who carry self-blame (the gateway to guilt) have greater amounts of inflammatory markers known as *cytokines*, which are known to contribute to a huge range of chronic disease states, in their blood.[1]

Several years ago, a dear friend of mine was diagnosed with leukemia. Within a week of finishing a course of chemotherapy, he experienced an aggressive flare-up of the cancer, and his doctors ended up recommending a bone marrow transplant.

The doctor who was leading his transplant, it turned out, had done extensive studies at the Chernobyl nuclear site, looking at the health impacts of radiation. He studied how some people develop aggressive, treatment-resistant cancers, while others go through chemo and go on to thrive for many years afterward. What he found was that emotions played a *huge* role in disease progression and recovery. His theory was that guilt mutates our cells and genes in a way that weakens immune function and the entire mind-body system. Oddly enough, my friend was someone who struggled with a huge amount of guilt throughout his life.

We often use guilt unconsciously as a way of continuing the same bad behavior. If you feel guilt about something, your mind takes this as a sign that you're "not all that bad." Feeling bad about what happened creates a certain separation from it, giving you a subtle way to continue the same behaviors and stay stuck in the same conditioned mind-sets.

You have two better choices here: (1) stop feeling guilty and just do whatever you want to do and accept the consequences, or (2) stop thinking about it and just change the way you're behaving. If you did either of those things, you would come back to the present moment in a place of acceptance. But we don't do that. Instead, we keep repeating the same behavior and feeling guilty about it. The cycle sounds something like this: *I did something bad, but I feel bad about it, so I'm not actually that bad, so let me just keep doing it.* This is what it looks like to be totally stuck in the past, cut off from your own vitality, potentiality, and feelings. Let me make that clear: too much guilt leads to disconnection and detachment from one's own heart and feelings. I see this all the time with perfectionists: they're trapped in a toxic loop of self-directed anger, frustration, blame, and guilt. I can recall how much this cycle was running me prior to the silence retreat. It still rears its ugly head from time to time, though not nearly as much as before. Perfectionists are people who are angry at themselves, but the anger is very suppressed and submerged. It manifests itself as being frustrated internally and quick to cast a silent judgment on oneself and others. Eventually, when there's this much toxicity inside, you have to either release it by blaming others or internalize the blame so much that you shut off from other people. This is a surefire way to have zero energy, creating not even a lukewarm life but a dead life.

Have you ever noticed that perfectionists aren't very creative? You don't want a perfectionist at the head of your innovation lab. They get things done, but they're not very good at generating new solutions and possibilities. A perfectionist just doesn't have the energy, clarity, or mental space to play with ideas or come up with anything new because too much of their mental energy is being consumed by the past. They may become successful, but they pay a big price for their success: chronic stress, physical health problems, anxiety and depression, isolation, and ultimately burnout.

Emotions of the Future: The Fear Spectrum

If you've been saying to yourself, "That doesn't sound like me," pay attention now. If you're not someone who spends most of your time stuck in the past, it's because you spend most of your time stuck in the future.

Thoughts of the future bring with them the fear spectrum of emotion, which also starts small and slowly builds up. It might initially sound like *I don't know, I'm not sure, But what if . . . ?* It begins with doubt and insecurity, not trusting oneself, which flows into worry, which flows into fear. When fear continues, it becomes chronic anxiety and ultimately panic attacks. It moves from the subtlest forms of self-doubt that you're not even conscious of all the way to needing medication to be calm enough to function in your daily life. All of these emotions stem from a negative apprehension of the future; the only difference is the intensity. You might be worried about a presentation you have to give at work tomorrow or doubting your ability to succeed in your new business. At a certain point, the worry snowballs so much that you're not sleeping well, or oversleeping; you can't think straight, and you can't focus on what you're doing. You start shrinking back in order to protect yourself and acting from a place of self-preservation, creating even more insecurity and doubt. This is the vicious cycle of the fear spectrum.

Our minds are like this! They're a pinball machine shooting back and forth endlessly between yesterday and tomorrow. The price we pay for this exhausting journey is the quality of the moment right in front of us.

From Phase 1, which is doubt and insecurity, you move into Phase 2: full-blown fear. This is when past memories are being powerfully triggered. You get flung back into the past and start to open old files in the mind that may be similar, or perhaps only vaguely related, to the imagined future you're worrying over. You'll remember that one time you got fired or racked up some debt, or the first date that went horribly. You justify and strengthen your fear by using examples from the past. You're no longer in a creative, flexible mind-set; you're in a place of avoidance and damage control. Notice that this fear cycle is draining the excitement and energy out of the new relationship, the new business venture, or any other opportunity or possibility that you wanted to invite into your life. When the fear becomes thick enough, you hit Phase 3: anxiety and panic. Internally, you're on total shutdown, lockdown mode. The fear extends beyond the specific situation to color everything in your life. You become plagued with unease and the constant sense of "something is wrong."

Notice how connected these emotions of the past and future are. What you need to see is that underneath the emotions of the future are always the emotions of the past. That's why Vedanta says that the root of all thought (even thoughts about the future) is *smriti*, the past. If someone comes to me complaining that they have anxiety, I know that 99 percent of the time, what we're really going to be working on is unexpressed anger. That person might be anxious about the direction of their career, but that's only what's in their conscious mind. That's only the tip of the iceberg. Beneath the surface level of awareness, the past and the emotions of the past are driving these fears. Underneath the anxiety and self-doubt, there is anger. Often it's anger toward themselves for the mistakes they've made and the ways they've failed to live up to their own expectations. There's self-blame and self-judgment that's causing them not to trust in their ability to create the life they want. The self-blame is a huge open file that's triggering hundreds of other related files, generating negative thoughts and feelings around the future. The simple truth is that what we focus on, we create more of in our lives. It's a basic law of attraction. But when we can understand, recognize, and address the deeper roots of the problem in the unconscious mind, the thoughts and emotions in the conscious mind naturally shift. This is the whole premise of psychotherapy. Change the direction of the iceberg at the base, and the surface will naturally follow.

Do you see how crazy brilliant and crazy insane this whole game is? Our minds are like this! They're a pinball machine shooting back and forth endlessly between yesterday and tomorrow. The price we pay for this exhausting journey is the quality of the moment right in front of us. It might not seem like much to you right now, but if you add up all the moments of regret or guilt or worry, you'll see how much of your life is being wasted. Add up the numbers: How much of your day are you wasting on something you can't change? Turn that into your week, then your month, then your year. This is where your precious energy, your life force, is going: not toward the things you want to build and create, not to the people and activities you love, not to your well-being, but to a past and future that are only real inside your own mind.

EXERCISE: Identifying Your Emotional Programming

Stop for a moment and go back to the exercise you did at the end of the last chapter. We're now going to finish filling in the last two columns. Looking over the items you wrote in the first column, ask yourself what specific positive or negative emotions each thought generates. Label the feelings, and be as specific as you can: joy, love, excitement, anger, frustration, insecurity, anxiety. Whatever it is, write it down in the third column. In column four, write down whether each item is related to the past, the future, or the now (now meaning not "recently" or "ongoing" but in this exact moment). Write a *P* for past, *F* for future, and *N* for now.

Look at how much time you're spending in the past and the future! Almost everything you think about is related to either one or the other. Which is more dominant for you? Do you tend to get stuck in anger, guilt, and regret over the past or anxiety and worry about the future? When you add it all up, how much of your time and energy is going into this? It's draining your energy faster than you can imagine, and this is only the surface, above-the-water level of the iceberg. Can you imagine what's going on in the base?

What's Unreal Is Not

There's a famous verse of the Bhagavad Gita, the seminal 700-verse Vedic scripture, that reads, "What's real *is*, and what's unreal *is not*." The unreal *was* and *will be*, but it never *is*. This is a bit of a mouthful, I know, but as abstract and esoteric as these words sound, they contain a very practical truth: *The past and future are not real.* They are not "reality" in the same way that the present moment is. You can never change them for the simple reason that they don't exist outside of your own mind!

What does it even mean to say that? The future is only our imagination of what our reality should and could be. It's a fantasy. And what we think of as past is only stored-up memories—memories that are colored by our own perspectives to begin with and highly likely to change and fade over time. A memory is nothing more than our own account of what happened, and it can never be an accurate account. Scientific studies on eyewitness testimony show that the same exact event is remembered radically differently by the different people who were there.[2] Eyewitness accounts are so notoriously inaccurate that they often interfere with legal proceedings. I can't tell you how many times as a prosecutor

I had four witnesses who saw the same thing, and each one gave a different story and pointed to a different person. That's when I started to realize that what we call "memory" is not the truth of a situation.

Even if you think you're recalling something clearly, at this moment it only exists in your mind, so it's not real. It never *is*. It doesn't exist. It's dead and gone, like a dream. While you're dreaming, the dream is real for you. Even a few moments after you wake up from a dream about someone chasing you, your heart is still beating fast, and your legs are tied up in the sheets as if you were trying to run away. It feels very real while it's happening, but within moments of when it ends, you're left feeling disoriented and unsure. Soon, the dream fades into a memory. Sometimes you wake up and you don't even remember what happened; you have only a vague idea that you might have had a dream that wasn't so good. A few hours later, the dream is totally gone. It no longer exists, just as it didn't exist before you dreamed it.

If you look at your life, at what happened yesterday and what happened a month ago, those things don't exist anymore, but they're dictating what does exist for you in the present. Maybe your mother or father abandoned you when you were young or a career that you put all your hopes and dreams into never worked out. While you were living it, it was very real and it was creating an impact. Then, after a certain amount of time has passed, it's still here with you. At some point you have to wake up and realize that it was a dream. It was the past. It's dead. It's gone. It does not exist now, and in this sense, it is not real. You learned a lesson, and now it's gone. Now you have a new moment to begin again. By holding on to what happened and making it real in your mind, by rehearsing the story again and again, always reminding yourself that "this happened to me," you make yourself a victim, and you give the past even more power. In this moment, you're operating from the power of the past, not the power of now.

Leaving the past behind is a choice that's always available to us. Some of the most celebrated leaders and visionaries in history survived unspeakable injustice and trauma, and they went on to live incredible lives. What happened to them was real when it happened, and it shaped who they are, but in order to move forward with their lives, they made the decision to live right now. Do you think Nelson Mandela spent his whole 27 years in jail being angry and resentful about the horrific injustices that he had experienced? No. He accepted the past and chose to do what he could in the present to create change. But we don't even have to look at these rare exceptions. There are people right under your nose, including yourself, who have many times picked up, dropped the past, and embraced the present to create an amazing future. One of them is Anthony Ray Hinton, an Alabama man who spent 30 years on death row for a crime he didn't commit. Shortly after being released from prison in April of 2018, he told ABC News, "Bitterness kills the soul. I cannot hate because my Bible teaches me not to hate. . . . What would it profit me to hate?"[3]

At some point you have to wake up and realize that it was a dream. It was the past. It's gone. Now you have a new moment to begin again.

What's real is what you have right now in front of you. Why get angry about what didn't work out? Why get angry about the boyfriend or girlfriend or mother or father who mistreated you? All of these things that stick to you are such a waste of time, effort, and, most of all, life force. You're spending so much of this precious moment back there reliving the pain again. Even if you're reliving the glories of the past, it is still a waste of this present moment.

One of the things that's so beautiful about Vedanta is that it looks at the mind from a holistic perspective, free from judgments of good and bad, positive and negative. We're not just chasing the positive and running away from the negative here. Vedanta tells us that positive and negative co-exist in life. Both are a part of life; one enhances, gives recognition and value to, the other. We value the positive because of the negative. Thinking too much about the past and future, even in a positive sense, takes your focus away from what's available to you right now. The positive expectations you create around the future also tend to lead to disappointment, which turns into regret—and there you are, stuck in the past again! If you were hoping to make $100,000 from a new business venture and you got $90,000, I'm willing to bet that you won't be focused on the success of the $90,000. You'll be focusing on what you should or could have done to get $100,000 or $110,000. This is how disappointment begins the downward spiral of regret, guilt, blame, and frustration—and down the rabbit hole we go.

The endless cycle of past and future thinking is a part of the basic nature of the mind, but that doesn't mean you're condemned to repeat it forever. The first way to break free is to do what you're doing right now: becoming aware of the fact that you're stuck in the cycle and knowing that your precious mental energy is going toward something that's fundamentally not real.

Second, you need to wake up to the price you're paying for being stuck in the past. Really look at what it's costing you. Somewhere, you are remaining in a fog. You're operating under the assumption that it's valuable, that it's working for you to stay in the past. But if you're being honest with yourself, you'll see that it's not! It's killing you. The brain likes the past because it's familiar and safe. But when we recognize how much it's hurting us to stay in the past, we learn our lesson. That flips our energy upward. Don't judge yourself for doing this—just realize that it's going on, accept it, and be grateful that you're taking steps to create change. When you change your mind-set from judgment to gratitude, your energy soars. This is what starts to break the pattern. The tools and techniques you'll learn about later in the book—breathwork, Vedic meditation, daily embodied practices, and mind-set shifts—can also help to recenter the mind in the present. But for now, the most important thing is to really take a good look at the way your internal world functions. We have to understand our own operating system before we can upgrade it.

The way to change your perception of the past is to remember two key things:

1. The past is nothing more than a dream.

2. Though you may not see it now, what happened in the past has served you in some way.

First, when you treat the past like a dream—when you really realize *it's gone, it's over, it's done*—you free yourself from the weight of it. Second, you have to realize that this is how it *had* to be. There is a greater plan for your life than you can possibly imagine. Don't judge yourself. It had to be this way for your greater good. Today you may or may not see it, but one day you will. Most of the time, you can only connect the dots looking backward, not forward. This is when you develop a sense of faith and an ability to see life from a broader context. I won't risk using the G-word here, but just know that there is *so* much to be gained from having faith in the unseen.

If you can move with the trust that there is a bigger plan, that things had to be this way, then you invite self-acceptance, self-love, self-compassion into your life. You reduce your negative self-judgments. You start to operate from a deep place of compassion, not only for yourself but also for those who may knowingly or unknowingly have hurt you.

Returning to the Now

Holding a broader vision of our lives helps us to return to the expansiveness of the present moment. This is the primary purpose of Vedanta: to teach us how to live a full, vibrant life, fully absorbed in the here and now. The moment we get out of the past and future where we're stuck and anchor the mind back in the present, we transcend the rigid box of conditioned thinking and dip into the ocean of pure consciousness—that field of energy and intelligence that is the substratum of life itself. When you dive into that ocean, you rinse off the limitedness, tightness, and contraction along with the anger, regret, fear, worry, and blame. It's like bathing under a waterfall. You enter this very wide state of mind called the present moment. You experience an explosion of energy.

Eckhart Tolle didn't invent the "power of now." The power of the present has been talked about for thousands of years in the Indian wisdom tradition. The Vedas have always described it as something that's innate to our existence. We were born with that power. As children we lived completely in the present. The power in our voice, in our gaze, and in our smile was unbounded. The real spiritual journey is the journey home to that place of power within ourselves. How do we get there? The Vedic system offers a road map filled with foolproof tools, techniques, and wisdom that provide the essential *how* for reconnecting with the power of now.

CHAPTER 6

The Mindfulness Trap

It amazes me that the one part of us that impacts everything in our lives more than any other—our own mind—comes with no instruction manual. It's critical to every single thing that we do, and yet no one has taught us how it really works or how to optimize its functions. Learning to deal with what's going on in the space between our ears is one of our biggest obstacles and longest journeys in life.

After everything we've just discussed, I'm sure you agree that you need tools to stop the incessant chatter of the frontal cortex and begin deleting the old, unneeded files from your memory. And with all the chaos going on not only inside our own minds but in our outside world today, the need for effective tools to deal with our minds has only increased. As rapidly as we're innovating and evolving, we're also becoming more disconnected from ourselves and others. There's so much anxiety to do and to achieve more and more, and the rapid pace at which the world is changing creates even more pressure to keep up. What's built today is already obsolete tomorrow. What's influential now is forgotten a year from now. The shelf life of our accomplishments keeps shortening along with our attention spans. What we've internalized from all this is the notion that if we're not keeping up, we're falling behind.

This pressure is so relentless that the deeper layers of the mind are not able to rest. Technology is a huge part of the problem: we're so connected to our devices that our minds never turn off. Checking our iPhones is the last thing we do at the end of the day and the first thing we do when we wake up in the morning, and the in-between, it isn't much better. Sleep has become an elusive phenomenon as our minds get more tightly wound. Constant overthinking, planning, and strategizing are so normal to us that we can't stop, even when we're trying to rest.

"Focus" sounds great. But how many of us really have the ability to focus on something sitting right in front of us for more than a few moments, much less something as subtle as the breath?

What's missing is rest and relaxation for the mind—and one place we can find it is in meditation. You're probably familiar with mindfulness meditation, which is one of the more popular meditation techniques in the West today. There are many benefits to this practice, and it's an excellent entry point into meditation. But as anyone who's tried it will tell you, the early stages of the practice itself are not very relaxing! One reason for this is what you just read above. We have never been trained at home or in school to deal with the incessant activity of our mind. We have never been educated in the art of relaxing. Mindfulness can actually do the opposite of resting the mind. It trains your attention muscles through focus and monitoring of thought, This has its own value, but you don't come to a place of calm restfulness until you reach the more advanced stages of the practice. As we'll see, there is an easier way to quiet and rest the mind almost immediately through effortless meditation, but first let's look at some of the opportunities and challenges of mindfulness practice that's become such a popular way of dealing with the mind.

What Mindfulness Is (and Isn't)

What are we really talking about when we talk about *mindfulness*? The word is used all the time and in every possible context (mindful eating, mindful sex, mindful investing, mindful parenting), but we often have only a vague sense of what it means. Mindfulness is defined as a "focused, nonjudgmental awareness of the present moment," cultivated most commonly through the practice of focusing one's attention on the breath.

Let's break that definition down for a moment: "Focus" sounds great. It's what you're looking for by turning to mindfulness in the first place. It's because you can't focus as much as you want, because your mind is wandering all over the place and you feel stressed, that you turn to mindfulness. But how many of us really have the ability to focus on something sitting right in front of us for more than a few moments, much less something as subtle as the breath? After all, it's not like there was ever a class in school on how to focus. I think you can see the difficulty in mindfulness if you have not practiced it before. At some level focus is a *prerequisite* for the practice of mindfulness and it's also the result you're looking for. This is like asking what came first, the chicken or the egg. That's our first challenge with this practice.

The second requirement of mindfulness is being "nonjudgmental." This is another mountain to climb. How many of us can honestly say that we're able to observe anything, let alone our own minds, without judgment? From the age of two onward—the time when our intellect begins to develop—we have a basic human tendency to judge something as soon as we see, hear, taste, or touch it. So let's look at how this plays out when you practice mindfulness meditation: here you are, sitting down to practice mindfulness, and just in the act of preparing to sit down, you feel resistance come up. The fact that there's resistance means you already have some judgment around it. Then you notice some thoughts, and you judge yourself for having those thoughts. Even if you don't judge the actual content of the thoughts, you judge yourself because you're "not supposed to be thinking." So then you tell yourself, "Don't judge"—another intellectual command, more frontal cortex activity. This may happen even if you've been practicing for some time. Then you start to ask yourself, *Why is my mind still so crazy after all this time of practicing mindfulness?* It keeps snowballing from there. I'm not saying this has to happen, but it is the natural tendency of the mind—yet undoing this tendency was the reason you went looking for mindfulness in the first place. So, once again, we find ourselves in a position where being nonjudgmental is the prerequisite as well as the result.

The third aspect of mindfulness practice is "awareness of the present moment," which brings us right back to the same challenge. Being mindful means being aware. Being aware is being present. The purpose of mindfulness is to be in the present moment, to bring the mind into the now, to increase awareness. And again, at some level the prerequisite of the practice is also the same: to be aware and present. How do you keep your mind in the present? By becoming aware of the breath, which is in the present moment, which is exactly the thing we "can't do." For many people, it's a vicious cycle that only creates a sense of struggle.

The Catch-22 of Mindfulness

Do you see the problem here? The methodology of mindfulness is interconnected with the outcome. We talk about mindfulness as a technique—a set of tools for becoming more aware—and also as a goal in itself. In order to become mindful, you need a certain degree of mindfulness to begin with. It's a catch-22. I am not telling you not to practice mindfulness, nor am I suggesting, if you practice mindfulness, that the practice has not served you. Instead, I am suggesting that there is an easier and faster way to meditate and become more mindful.

But first, let's separate the techniques from the goal for a moment. The techniques of modern mindfulness practice are a specific set of tools, derived from 2,500-year-old Buddhist principles (which can be traced back even further to the Vedanta!), that have been distilled and repackaged for Western consumption. The primary tool is *focused attention*, the practice of sustaining one's focus on a single object, typically the breath. Then there's *mental monitoring*, the process of observing one's own physical or mental activity and labeling it: "I'm sitting, sitting," "breathing, breathing," "thinking, thinking," "worrying, worrying." The basic idea is to focus your awareness on the breath or the mental activity and to gently bring your mind back each time you notice that it's wandered. And boy, does the mind wander. In mindfulness practice, just as in daily life, our attention is constantly being pulled away from the here and now to everywhere. This, our habituated mind, is what makes the practice "difficult."

If you've ever seen a Woody Allen movie, you know that his character is constantly caught up in some imaginary catastrophe. What mindfulness essentially does is ask Woody Allen to be calm, quiet, and nonjudgmental. It asks him to observe himself from a detached, neutral perspective, which goes against his very nature.

The mind-wandering is where the real struggle comes in. Think of it this way: It's as if you were walking around all day, every day, with a Woody Allen character in your head—a constant negative commentary on everything you think, say, and do. I'm sorry to say that, if you could hear your own internal dialogue, you'd find that, at some level, you really are walking around with a Woody Allen in there. We all are.

If you've ever seen a Woody Allen movie, you know that his character is constantly caught up in some imaginary catastrophe. What mindfulness essentially does is ask Woody Allen to be calm, quiet, and nonjudgmental. It asks him to observe himself from a detached, neutral perspective, which goes against his very nature.

We are often completely absorbed in our own problems—of course we can't see ourselves clearly! The only way for us to find peace of mind is to get help from someone outside of our own head: a friend or a therapist. The therapist provides the neutral perspective necessary for us to observe ourselves clearly. But imagine just talking to yourself instead of to a therapist. Now all you're doing is adding more neurosis, more judgment, more confusion, on top of what's already there! You sitting in a therapy session with yourself is not going to help you reach greater clarity. Instead, you're simply going to get more worked up. This is what often happens when we practice mindfulness. We're asking the mind that is already unfocused, judgmental, and caught up in the past or future to be a wise and compassionate Buddha. What we need is a tool outside of the mind to transform the habits of the mind.

When I look at the current conversation around mindfulness, what I see is Woody Allen trying to calm himself down and often getting even more stuck in his own thoughts. What I *don't* see is a way of becoming mindful that's fast and simple at the starting gate for most people.

Mindfulness vs. Vedic Meditation

Based on years of experience teaching Vedic meditation to thousands of people—but not mindfulness as we know it in the West—I've come to believe that, while mindfulness has brought a lot of value to a lot of people, it is not meditation. Instead, it is a rather difficult entry point *to* meditation. In the Vedic tradition, meditation is defined as a process of finding restful alertness. It's a tool for *deeply resting* the *entire* mind so that we naturally operate with greater awareness. By that definition, again, I have to say that mindfulness is not meditation. Perhaps it was what we needed 50 years ago when it was first brought to the West, but today, we need to step up the game. We need something both deeper and simpler than the ability to focus, wouldn't you agree? What's really missing—what we need over and above sharpened focus and attention—is the ability to deeply rest every level of the mind and memory while effortlessly expanding our awareness. The solution to optimizing the functions of the mind must address the entire iceberg, from the top to the bottom. Any technique that addresses only the tip is incomplete.

I've been a Vedic meditation teacher for over 30 years. I've traveled all over the world instructing thousands of people in ancient meditative techniques. I meet so many people who need and want so badly to calm the chatter and soothe the trauma in their minds. They turn to mindfulness as a solution and don't "succeed" at it. They'll tell me that they've given up on the whole idea, and they're trying some new diet or workout or sleeping pill instead. I find this heartbreaking. I can't tell you how many times I've said, "No, no, no, go back to meditation! Please!"

If the rishis and the Buddha himself could hear the way we talk about mindfulness today, I think they'd have a big belly laugh. Why are we working the mind so hard when the whole point is to relax it? What are we doing adding more mental effort on top of all the crap that's already there? What I've observed is that modern mindfulness is a difficult, arduous, and incomplete journey. When mindfulness was first brought to the West, only a tiny piece of the full practice was introduced. Today, I'm happy to see that many mindfulness practitioners are slowly adding other elements, like chanting or precepts, to the practice of mindfulness. I'm not denying the value of mindfulness on its own, but I'd like to suggest that there are faster, easier techniques for reducing stress and becoming more present.

These techniques aren't some new hack or innovation. Instead, they're rooted in the most ancient origins of meditation itself. We'll discuss this in depth in Chapter 8, but for now, let's continue to look at some of the common pitfalls and limitations of mindfulness practice as we know it.

The Power of NOW, but HOW?

I believe wholeheartedly in the "power of now," but the bigger question is, *How?* How to be more mindful? How to bring the mind back into the present moment? From what I've seen, mindfulness isn't providing any easy, practical answers to these questions.

I believe wholeheartedly in the "power of now,"
but the bigger question is, How?

As much as everyone likes to talk about mindfulness, you'd be surprised at how few people are actually able to do it until they reach advanced stages of practice. I've heard more stories about "failed attempts" at mindfulness than you could possibly imagine. In the long run, it's not a failed attempt. Everything makes some difference, but the practice fails to have its intended effect because most people lose patience and give up. The message I hear is: *I want to learn how to be more calm and present, but mindfulness doesn't really work for me.* Most people give up on mindfulness when their thoughts refuse to settle down, and others are too intimidated by the practice to even try it. People who have been practicing regularly for years tell me that they still struggle to keep their focus on the breath for more than a minute. Others say that sitting and being present to their thoughts somehow leaves them feeling even more stressed, anxious, and agitated than when they started.

The dialogue around mindfulness promises so much—radiant health, inner peace, success in business and relationships—but the reality is that most people can't sit still and focus their attention on the breath for more than 30 seconds; therefore, few manage to ever achieve these miraculous benefits. Shortly before I wrote this book, I was giving a lecture at a company that had invested heavily in bringing mindfulness practices to its employees. During the lecture, I did a short exercise with the group during which I asked them to consciously bring to mind, without judgment, a stressful situation or event that was currently going on at home or with their work. After a few moments of simply recalling and being present with the stressful situation, I asked how they were feeling. The response was what you'd expect: increased heartbeat, racing thoughts, negative emotions, elevated body temperature, a sense of contraction, and a racing internal dialogue. Then I asked them to spend a few moments just sitting and focusing on their breath and feelings. After 10 minutes of me talking had passed, I turned and asked, "How do you feel now? Are you all present and listening? Do you feel less stressed? Are you more in the present moment? Where is your attention?" Across the room, almost all 200 people raised their hands to indicate that they still felt stressed. There was still the lingering residue of stress from the event that had been brought to their mind. They were less present and less attentive to the session. They were still caught up in the adrenaline response going on in their bodies. Then I asked the obvious questions. "The stress from the event is an open file in the background of your mind. What are you going to do with it? How will you close the file? It's using up your energy. How do you shut it down?" Nobody had an answer—including the lead mindfulness trainer! Sitting there watching the breath for another 20 minutes was not an option in the middle of the workday.

I was sitting in a room full of more than 200 avid mindfulness practitioners. Most of these people had a daily practice of at least 30 minutes. Here they were being mindful of what was creating stress for them, but they didn't know what to do about it. "Being mindful" did not relieve the stress or make them more present, nor were they able to experience the event free from their negative judgments. When I say that mindfulness as we know it is an incomplete process, that's what I mean: it may make us more aware of where the mind is stuck, but it doesn't necessarily help us to get unstuck.

Why is that? What exactly is going on here? The truth is that mindfulness, as a particular set of techniques for increasing awareness, is hard. *Really* hard. It has an incredible amount of value, but it requires time, effort, discipline, and work—internal work, which most of us don't have time for or feel that we're able to do. It works optimally in the setting for which it was designed: meaning sitting in a monastery, without worldly pressures and demands to perform and achieve at high levels. But in our modern lives, things are a little more complicated.

Even mindfulness teachers and avid practitioners describe the practice using a language of struggle. In the kindest tone, you will hear Jon Kabat-Zinn, founder of Mindfulness-Based Stress Reduction, who is often credited with bringing the practice to the West, describe the process as an uphill climb. "Mindfulness requires effort and discipline for the simple reason that the forces that work against our being mindful . . . are exceedingly tenacious," he writes in his book *Wherever You Go, There You Are*. He adds, "This process doesn't magically happen by itself. It takes energy." Notice that he's saying that the practice requires energy to begin with. Unfortunately, it's the lack of energy and a tired mind that make us want to meditate in the first place. Lucky for us, there are magical tools available in Vedanta.

Mindfulness experts admit that it can take years of hard work in order to get anywhere—but who has that kind of time? Who can expend that kind of effort and energy? I came across one account from a mindfulness teacher who said that after practicing for more than 10 years, she still "fails 90 percent of the time." Again, stop and notice the vocabulary being used here: *Effort. Fail.* I'm exhausted just thinking about it!

You know from what we've discussed so far that the mind functions optimally on the principle of *effortlessness*. It's about less mental work and activity so that we can experience the present moment more directly, allowing intuition and insight to arise. That's the benefit. But with mindfulness, until you're very advanced, you don't reach this goal. You stay in this place of "more mental work."

How did we get it so backwards?

Skimming on the Surface of the Mind

The reason that mindfulness is creating more mental effort and less ease is simple: it's because it's keeping us on the surface level of the mind, where all of our thinking is going on.

These techniques of focused attention and mental monitoring are controlled mind functions occurring on the tip of the iceberg, the tiny sliver of consciousness that we're aware of and have some say over. Like rational thinking and strategizing, they activate the brain's frontal cortex. Scientists studying mindfulness have found that the practice actually *increases* the volume and density of the frontal cortex. This has the benefit of enhancing functions like attention and emotion regulation, decision-making, learning, surface-level memory, and cognitive control. But the downside of these more narrow practices is that they restrict our awareness to the surface of the ocean. They cut us off from the more powerful base of the iceberg. They separate us from the ocean itself. Mindfulness practices restrict your ability to reach the deeper states of conscious, including flow states, which require the quieting down of the frontal cortex.

When you practice mental monitoring, you're only monitoring what you can control, which is the very top layer of thought. It's the frontal cortex that's engaged, not the whole brain. That's like swimming on the surface of the water, looking out at the oncoming waves, and yelling to yourself, "Three-foot wave!" "Four-foot wave!" "Two-foot distance between waves!" You're more aware of the waves on the surface, sure, but you're missing the depth, breadth, and power of the ocean below you. You might learn to better ride the waves, but underneath the surface—in the memory bank, the deeper levels of intellect and perception, and the subconscious—those thoughts and feelings that are creating the waves in the first place are completely unaffected. These submerged activities are exhausting your mind and causing your consciousness to contract with more fear, agitation, and reactivity.

When you practice mental monitoring, you're only monitoring the very top layer of thought. That's like swimming on the surface of the water and yelling to yourself, "Three-foot wave! Four-foot wave!" You're missing the depth, breadth, and power of the ocean below you.

Fundamentally, what these techniques are doing is trying to *solve the problems of the mind on the level of the mind*. We're trying to fix the glitch using the bugged computer itself instead of getting an outside technician. While it's possible to do that, it's more difficult than it needs to be.

Focusing your attention on surface-level mental disturbances can also have the unwelcome side effect of amplifying them. Have you ever noticed that? When new practitioners go on their first mindfulness retreat, they're often surprised to find that instead of feeling a sense of peace and calm, they're overwhelmed with very intense emotions. It's not that those emotions weren't there before, but now you're suddenly becoming very aware of them—often along with feelings of judgment. For instance, you might be practicing mindfulness and become aware of the fact that you have a lot of anxiety around being alone. So you observe, and repeat to yourself, "anxious, anxious, anxious." On a subtle level, you're adding fuel to the anxiety. The thoughts don't disperse; instead, you hold on to them even more. Rather than allowing yourself to fully experience the feeling of anxiety and then let it go, you fixate on it. Just noticing the thought and telling yourself that it's there is not enough to make it shift or disperse. Remember what happened to that corporate group of mindfulness practitioners. They became aware of their stress and anxiety, but they couldn't do anything about it. They walked into their next meeting with the old files open and the stress in full swing.

The Zombie Effect

In the long run, too much attention regulation and monitoring can actually dampen our vibrancy and vitality. If we're creating internal "discipline" instead of pure awareness, it can numb our emotions and shut down the deeper levels of intuition and creative force, bringing a certain level of disconnect and dullness over time. We are meant to live, experience, and express our inner life, not just observe or control it. Have you ever noticed that some long-term mindfulness practitioners don't look so lively and energetic? Perhaps they are monitoring and labeling life rather than living it. This is like the difference between reading a recipe for a delicious cake versus just eating it.

There can be something a bit placid and sedated in the expression of life and passion of long-term mindfulness practitioners. I have seen many of them sitting around and talking about thriving, but they don't *exude* thriving. There's no passion in their voices! Many people see this, and when they come to me, they worry that mindfulness will take away their edge, that it will dampen their passion and creativity. What can I say? A dulling effect can and does happen when you're caught up in monitoring rather than living.

It's my belief that we are not supposed to monitor everything in life. We are just supposed to live. Too-active monitoring is what numbs and dumbs us. It slows the creative flow from a rushing river to a tiny trickle. Just look at someone like the Dalai Lama: he's not hyperfocused or trying to monitor anything. He is the most natural, free human being you could possibly imagine. The Dalai Lama is simply existing as himself. He exudes this abundance of happiness, peace, and confidence without even trying. His laugh is enough to make even the most cynical person smile! I notice these qualities in Sri Sri also. He has abundant stamina and energy. He travels all over the world meeting with hundreds of thousands of people, greeting everyone with a joy and deep connection that's absolutely electric. This is what we're really looking for from our practice—not to walk around like zombies but to be natural, lively, vibrant human beings.

If you're any kind of a spiritual practitioner, including a mindfulness practitioner, the big question to ask yourself is this: Do you feel more lively, energetic, inspired, and free? Or are you more subdued, contained, and seemingly in control? If your life and your energy are becoming bigger and more exuberant, then keep going! Rock on. But if this liveliness isn't showing up in your life, then I think you should consider looking for something different. If you aren't feeling more dynamic and vibrant, then there's something off in whatever you're doing, whether it's called "mindfulness" or "yoga" or TM or any other thing.

The natural joy of the Dalai Lama reminds us that Buddhism in its full expression doesn't teach mindfulness in such a fragmented, isolated way. Focusing one's attention on the breath, labeling and monitoring thoughts and emotions, is just one aspect of the tradition that the West took away and repackaged. I don't think the Buddha himself sat around only focusing on the breath, monitoring and labeling his own mental activity, walking like a zombie. Buddhism has its roots in the Vedic tradition, and the Buddha practiced all the things that come out of Vedanta: the ethical precepts, the mind-set principles, the breathing techniques, and the energizing practices—everything you'll be learning throughout the rest of this book. In Eastern spiritual traditions, the practice of mindfulness was usually the natural result, the end point that included many other practices and techniques to bring not just peace and quiet but also vibrancy and power.

"No Mind," Not "More Mind"

Remember what I said at the beginning of this chapter: Mindfulness and Vedic meditation are not the same thing. In the Vedic tradition, meditation is not about maintaining your focus. It's the process of *loosening* your focus so that your mind can relax and your thoughts can naturally unwind, resulting in focus and clarity. The rishis say that there's no need to label or monitor your thoughts, and most importantly, you don't have to focus! The Sanskrit word for meditation is *dhyana—dhya* means "to focus, pay attention, or concentrate," and *na* is the negation of focus, attention, or concentration. It's a state of "no focus" or "open focus"—"no concentration" or "no mind," not "more mind"! This state of "no focus" is something we already do naturally. The mind naturally wanders and defocalizes when it needs to rest. Utilizing this natural tendency to expand our focus in the process of becoming mindful has far more value and requires much less effort than trying to harness focus. Whether we practice focused attention or "no focused attention," both roads ultimately lead to the same place. The difference is how long and arduous the journey will be.

Meditation, in the yogic sense, comes down to any practice or activity that guides the senses, along with the mind, into quieter states of awareness. Notice I used the words *natural* and *effortless*: not forced, not disciplined, not insisting. By using tools *outside* of the mind, we can simply allow the senses to go quiet so that the mind goes quiet. The way to quiet the senses is so simple: Let the mind drift, let it think, invite it to think, give it permission to do whatever it wants to do. Do nothing additional with your mind. Just be.

In the Vedic tradition, meditation is not about maintaining your focus. It's the process of loosening your focus so that your mind can relax and your thoughts can naturally unwind, resulting in focus and clarity.

Working mentally in order to quiet the mind is an oxymoron. You're trying so hard when the whole point is for the mind to not try at all. The point is to work less, think less, do less, and achieve more. Here's my advice to you: Stop trying! Stop working. Stop efforting, and stop controlling. Give your mind a break. You don't have to swim upstream. You don't have to cling to the riverbank for fear of being swept away by the current of thoughts and emotions. As the Beatles (who practiced Transcendental Meditation) said: "Turn off your mind, relax, and float downstream." The mind will naturally flow toward deeper, stiller waters if you simply allow it to.

When the mind relaxes and the thinking process unwinds—including the monitoring, labeling, and focusing—consciousness naturally expands. As we move beyond controlled thinking processes, the mind drops into deeper states of relaxation until the river merges with the ocean of pure awareness. From this place, life force shoots up. And again, when there's more energy, you are naturally aware, without even trying. We call this "effortless awareness." When the mind is relaxed, you are in the present moment. You don't have to "try" to be that way, you just are! It is your nature. Have you ever seen how alert and aware a newborn baby is? There's no *doing* in order to be aware; it's just a state of being. It's how we are born. It just gets covered with layers and layers of mental activity. Meditation is a practice of letting that drop so that who you are, awareness, can shine through. It's important to note that being mindful or aware is not an action, but rather our deepest nature. Peel back the layers of the mind and what remains is pure awareness.

Tools *outside of the mind* for increasing awareness were encoded in the Vedic texts thousands of years ago as part of a comprehensive road map for managing the mind. Controlled breathing practices and *dhyana* don't require months and years of hard work. You will see the benefits immediately. When I talk about breathing and meditation, I'm talking about the use of the breath as an exercise, not monitoring the breath. And I don't mean meditation in the sense of focusing attention with mental effort. The style of meditation that I teach and practice is a technique in Vedanta known as *Sahaj Samadhi* meditation, or "natural effortless" meditation. It's a simple, effective technique, closely related to Transcendental Meditation, in which the practitioner effortlessly "transcends" the controlled mind—the labeling, judging, thinking mind—to reach the state of pure awareness. We'll come back to this in Chapter 8.

But first, we start with the breath. As the ancient science of Vedanta—as well as modern neuroscience—shows, the breath directly impacts our mental state, but it's not a faculty of the mind. The breath travels not only on the surface of the mind but across the entire mind. It moves from the controlled mind, the intellect, and the memory through the subconscious and unconscious systems, as well as the ego, all the way down to the very source of all thought and emotion in the ocean of consciousness. We are using a physical process to create change on a mental level. There is a faster, simpler, effortless way to be not only mindful but also calm and energized. The secret is literally right under your nose: the breath. But it's not about monitoring the breath, it's about how you *use* the breath.

Part III

REBOOT

AND

RECHARGE

CHAPTER 7

The Secret of Life

What was the first thing you did when you came into the world? And what's the last thing you'll do when you leave this planet? The answer to both questions is right under your nose. The first thing you did was take a deep breath in, and it's certain that the last act of your life will be to breathe out. The breath is so obvious that we take it for granted, but stop to think about it a moment. Breathing is the most important thing you do on a daily basis. It is life itself. It is the one faculty that keeps you not only alive but moving and going after all that matters to you most. Surely something as critical to our existence as this must be more than a passive, mechanical function. And it is: Within the breath is the secret of life itself. It is the secret to changing the state of our thoughts, emotions, perception, and vitality. The only problem is that no one has ever taught us how to utilize its power.

The breath is the simplest and most effective tool we have for getting the mind unstuck. We just need to learn how to use it. It's mind-boggling to think that in the frantic rush of our demanding lives, we have forgotten how to breathe, and as a result we have cut ourselves off from our greatest source of power. How many times do you find yourself holding your breath during moments of stress? It happens so much that you're not even aware of it, but there's no doubt that it has a huge impact on your thoughts, emotions, and outlook.

Fortunately for us, the rishis knew that the key to mastering the mind was to raise our innate life force by introducing the natural rhythm of the breath. They understood that when life's stresses throw us off-balance, it creates chaotic rhythms within us, and we feel a sense of discomfort and discontent. The mind wavers, vacillating between worries about the future and the regrets of the past. We find that we are not fully alive or enjoying our lives in the present moment, here and now. Within the rishis' science of life enhancement, a specific set of techniques for tapping into the power of the breath is the most critical tool we've been given. The phenomenal thing about the breath is that it's a physical activity, like a workout, that anyone can do. It does not require any focus, concentration, manipulation of thoughts, or mental activity. Breathing is the fastest, simplest way to reduce stress and naturally shift the way you think, feel, and act. It's the master key to unlocking the potential of your entire system. When practicing breathing, you will be amazed at how quickly the time passes and the instant value you gain not only in energizing yourself but in becoming more present and aware.

The big ancient secret is this: *there is an "off" switch for the mind, and that switch is the breath.* The Vedic texts describe in astonishing detail what scientists have only recently "discovered": that the breath acts as a kind of control board for the nervous system. It is the one means we have to deactivate the stress response that arises from the *sympathetic nervous system* (the fight-flight-freeze system) and activate the *parasympathetic* nervous system—the rest, relax, and rejuvenate response. Using the breath alone, we can switch from the survival mode of the sympathetic system to the thriving mode of the parasympathetic system.

Stuck in Survival Mode

We spend most of our lives operating from the sympathetic system. While this system is a major energy hog, it's not inherently bad. In fact, it's critical to our ability to function in life. If you're being chased by a lion, that fight-or-flight response is going to save your life. But when the sympathetic switch gets stuck in the "on" position, then you respond to the smallest of things as if a lion were chasing you. In these moments, you're operating from the limbic brain, reacting from the negative past instead of responding with a clear, calm mind in the present. You're in a mind-set of resistance and avoidance, focusing on the negative and seeing from a glass-half-empty perspective, which we'll discuss more in Chapter 11. Your system is releasing powerful bursts of energy and hormones such as adrenaline to help you escape from the imaginary lion. In effect, you're burning through your life force.

Breathing is the fastest, simplest way to reduce stress and naturally shift the way you think, feel, and act. It's the master key to unlocking the potential of your entire system.

The problem here is that our biology hasn't caught up with our modern lives. We act as if we're being chased by a lion when we hear the ping of an email alert, realize we're a few minutes late for a meeting, get cut off in traffic, or read troubling news headlines. When we can't find our phones or our wallets, our systems register it as a threat to our survival. The brain is simply unable to distinguish between something that is really happening and something we've just imagined. In either case, the chemical reaction is one of fear. Before you even blink, thousands of chemical signals have been sent throughout the brain, kicking the nervous system into a state of high alert and triggering a cascade of physical responses (racing heart, sweaty palms, dilating pupils, tensing muscles, and fast, shallow breaths). This becomes another vicious cycle: something happens that triggers a negative thought, the thought creates an emotion, which creates a set of physical sensations, which generates a specific breathing pattern, which then re-creates similar thoughts. This is the cycle of what we call *karma*—"bondage to the past." We keep creating the same response over and over again. So how the hell do we turn it off?

Talking to yourself, telling yourself to calm down, won't change your thoughts and emotions. What you *can* change is your breathing. This is the golden key. The breath is the only part of the fight-or-flight response that we can control, so that's what we use to break out of the cycle. It's the one mechanism that is both sympathetic and parasympathetic. It's an automatic process, but you also have some control over it. It moves by itself if you don't pay attention to it, but you can also consciously manipulate it in order to reboot and rebalance the entire system.

The way it works is so simple. When you consciously change the pattern of your breath, you change what's going on in your mind. Whether you slow it down, speed it up, hold on to it, release it, suck it in fast, or thrust it out forcefully, if you change your breathing in some way, then you will change your thoughts and emotions. You shift the physical sensations that are being interpreted by your neurological system and giving rise to those mental responses. What we know is that the longer and smoother the breath, the fewer gaps there are in the breath, and thus the more aware, calm, controlled, and dynamic our mental faculties are. The longer you can retain the breath you've taken in, the more your thought processes shift toward the parasympathetic response—calmness and relaxation—which then changes your emotions. It also changes your physical sensations, which further change the messages firing in your synapses—a virtuous cycle!

When you breathe with the rhythm of relaxation, it sends a signal to the nervous system to shift into rest-and-relax mode. The adrenals stop pumping out stress hormones, heart rate decreases, blood pressure lowers, and the parasympathetic nervous system takes over.[1] With the physiological stress response turned off, negative thoughts and emotions begin to unwind. You then start conserving and even gaining energy. This isn't just a nice idea; it's a very real and powerful phenomenon. Research into the effects of yogic breathing practices like the ones described in the Vedas have shown how quickly and effectively they can break the cycle of stress by way of rebalancing the nervous system. Scientists studying Sudarshan Kriya, the series of yogic breathing techniques I've taught for the past three decades, have found that the practice lowers stress hormone levels, improves sleep quality, strengthens the immune system, and reduces or eliminates symptoms of anxiety, depression, PTSD, and addiction.[2] The breath acts like what herbalists call an *adaptogen*. It helps the body adapt better to stress so that physical and mental processes throughout the system can return to a state of harmony and homeostasis.

The Power of Prana

It all comes back to our innate energy. When we shut down the breath, we lose huge amounts of energy. Energy is low, the mind gets stuck in negativity, and the way we feel and act—and in turn, what we attract in life—reflects that state of low vibration. But when we come back to our natural breathing patterns, the whole system gets a recharge. Energy is high, we're in a positive state of thought and emotion, we act from a place of calm clarity, we are resilient in the face of challenges, and we create amazing things in our lives. Leaving it up to chance to decide that when we happen to feel good, we have good energy, and when we don't, we have bad energy, is foolishness. I see people leave their energy to circumstance, and then they wonder why they don't feel more in control of their lives. It's no mystery to me. It has been known for thousands of years how to quickly change the state of our minds and directly impact the state of our lives.

There's a simple but powerful saying in Vedanta: "Without life force, you are not alive." To the rishis, it's the most obvious thing in the world. But as modern people, we completely overlook this basic fact of how we function. We don't pay any attention to enhancing our life force through our breathing, and therefore we miss out on the most precious natural resource that's available to us. No matter where we are or what we're doing, the breath is always with us. It's like our own personal charging cable, conveniently accessible 24 hours a day, 7 days a week.

Breathing isn't about carbon dioxide and oxygen only. Otherwise you'd just slap an oxygen mask on your face and go about your day, and you'd be a total powerhouse.

We forget that the breath is literally what brings life into our system. The inhale is what gives us energy; it's what brings in *prana*. Between the two breaths through which we enter and exit the world, we take in millions of breaths. Each time we breathe, there is an amazing phenomenon happening: the in-breath brings in life force and distributes it throughout the system, while the out-breath releases what's no longer needed and detoxifies the mind and body. Think about it: When you're depressed, a deep sigh, which pushes so much stale air out of the body, gives you relief. When you're stressed, a long exhale helps you calm down by releasing whatever tension you're holding. There is something more than air that's released in the exhale: you breathe out because it gives room to the mind to take more in.

Breathing isn't about carbon dioxide and oxygen only. Otherwise you'd just slap an oxygen mask on your face and go about your day, and you'd be a total powerhouse. It's not that simple. There is something much deeper and more essential going on here. The breath has the ability to bring so much *Shakti,* so much vital energy, into the system, it's hard to even imagine until you've experienced it for yourself. You only need to charge up for a short period of time, and you'll have the battery power you need to keep you running through the day. A short time spent breathing reboots the entire system. Then, when you're fully charged, you're so much more vibrant and alive. You operate on a different level. For thousands of years, sages, shamans, monks, and yogis have been tapping this power, using the breath to turn down the volume of the thinking mind and expand their consciousness all the way to enlightenment.

One story in the Upanishads, one of the key texts of the Vedas, describes the mental faculties and the five senses fighting against each other to try to prove which one of them is the most important. Mind, breath, speech, hearing, smell, touch, and sight are all determined to prove their superiority in the human system. In order to determine who is the best of all, they decide to leave the body one by one to see who will be the most sorely missed. Hearing flees, but the body continues functioning as deaf, still enjoying all of its other functions. Sight leaves, and the body is blind, but it still goes on. Touch leaves, and the body is still alive and functioning. Even when the mind leaves (taking all the senses with it), the body goes on existing in an unconscious state. Finally, with the departure of the breath, the body starts dying. All of the other faculties lose their energy. Thus breath is crowned the highest faculty. Without the *prana* that's brought in through the breath, the system simply cannot function. Another story from the Upanishads compares the breath to a queen bee. In a beehive, the queen is the mother of nearly all of the thousands of other bees in the hive, and as the sole reproductive partner, she is single-handedly responsible for whether the bee colony thrives or not. As the story goes, when the queen bee flies away, all the other bees—meaning all of our other physical and mental faculties—fly away also. But when she sits, "all the other bees sit around her." The moral of both stories is this: the secret to controlling all of our faculties is controlling our breath.

Yoga master B. K. S. Iyengar says ignoring the use and development of the breath is like having a fortune locked in a bank account that you forget the password to. It's like sitting on top of a gold mine and begging for spare change! You're turning to espressos and green juices and SoulCycle classes for little hits of energy to keep you going, when the vast energy of the universe is accessible to you at every moment through this umbilical cord of the breath.

You might be thinking at this point that none of this applies to you, that you breathe just fine already, but thanks anyway. If you think you "don't need to work on your breathing," I'm here to tell you that you're wrong. The truth is that most of us use only around 30 percent of our lung capacity. That means your battery is only 30 percent charged! You're only using a third of your capacity to energize and a third of your capacity to release and detoxify. Most of us don't inhale fully, we don't exhale fully, and we hold our breath, cutting ourselves off from the source of energy. It's not difficult to learn how to breathe again, but it does require a little time and willingness on your end. Know that whatever time and energy you put in you will quickly gain back.

If you can just change your breath a little bit (which you can, trust me), then you can also change your state of mind and quality of life. Of course, I don't expect you to believe any of this until you've experienced it for yourself. It's almost impossible to imagine how much of a difference the breath can make before you have experienced it. After all, you just think of breathing as something you do all the time. It's as normal to you as blinking or eating or pooping. I've been teaching this stuff for almost three decades, and trust me, it's not always easy to get people on board. I feel like I'm trying to sell snow to an Eskimo when I tell a new corporate group, "Look, here's your breath, use it!" They will either look at me like I'm crazy, or they'll nod along vacantly while their eyes glaze over. Or they'll say, "What are you talking about? I'm breathing already. I don't need to learn that." So if you're feeling a little skeptical right now, that's fine. Try to hold your judgments for now. As we go on, you'll learn to develop an energy superpower that will support and empower you in everything you do in life.

Digging Deeper into the Breath-Emotion Connection

This connection between the breath and the mind ain't rocket science. It's a simple observation that anyone would make if they just took the time to look. Observing the breath reveals that specific emotions have always been attached to particular breathing patterns. We tell people to "just take a deep breath" when they need to calm down because we know that a deep, steady breath is connected to feelings of ease and peacefulness. There's a specific rhythm of breath for not only peacefulness but every single emotion we have as human beings. The breath influences the emotions, and the reverse is also true: the emotions impact the breath.

Back in ancient India, they didn't need fMRI scanners or EEG machines to prove that quality of breath is inextricably linked to quality of thought and emotion. The rishis methodically observed different breathing patterns to find what kinds of emotions, mental states, energy levels, and physical sensations were connected with those particular breathing patterns. Neuroscientists today are doing their own version of this in studies where they show people images designed to evoke certain emotions and then measure their breathing patterns throughout the process. What they've found is that when the participants view an image of a gun or a violent scene, their breath automatically shortens and tightens, but when they look at a butterfly or a baby laughing, their breath becomes deeper and more elongated.

Let's look at the breath in a state of anger. When rage starts to rise up, the breath moves in a very clear pattern: it's rapid, short and staccato. The temperature of the breath heats up, and the volume of air going in and out decreases. Because our breathing is intimately connected to our physical machinery, we also experience very specific bodily reactions: tightening and clenching in different areas, a racing heart, body temperature and blood pressure rising. The head contracts, and that contraction goes down into the neck and causes the nerves to throb. Anger also triggers specific parts of the brain that are very different from the brain areas that are activated when we're sad or relaxed or joyful, and this impacts the types of electromagnetic impulses being sent between neurons. Thoughts turn negative, outlook and perception go dark, and we experience the feeling of being "blinded" by the anger. It affects us even down to the level of DNA, and over time, it shortens our telomeres, the caps on the ends of our chromosomes that determine our health and longevity. When we're experiencing a lot of stress—which is almost always connected to negative emotions such as grief, fear, and frustration—we'll say things like *This past month was so stressful, I feel like I just aged five years.* On some level, we can sense what's going on within our anatomy.

My breathing was terrible before I learned how to use it. When I walked into Sri Sri's lecture as this uber-skeptical, high-octane lawyer thinking it was ridiculous to learn how to breathe, I could barely inhale for two seconds.

When we breathe with the rhythm of relaxation, on the other hand, feelings of peace, calm, and joy naturally arise. The mind returns to the present moment. The longer and deeper the breath, the more energy we have and the more mindful and aware we are naturally. This is our *natural* breath pattern—the way we breathed when we were children—but it's not the way we breathe most of the time as adults. The breath, like the mind, gets stuck. It's narrowed itself and tightened up. Look at your own breathing for a moment. Take a long, deep breath in and notice: Does your abdomen go in or out? For many people, the belly goes in and the shoulders and chest rise up—which is the very opposite of the way we naturally breathe. If you look at babies, you'll see that their abdomens go *out* as they breathe in. Part of the reason why children have so much energy is because they breathe in the most natural diaphragmatic rhythm. They bring in tons of energy through the inhale, and they release everything that's stuck on the exhale. As we get older and collect tension in the mind and body, the pattern reverses. We start holding stress and tension in our belly region, the area known in the Japanese tradition as the *hara*, the center of power in the body. When we flip this around, we naturally shift the state of the mind from dull and drained to expanded and uplifted.

The Breath Never Lies

I find so many secrets hidden in the breath. You'd be shocked at how much you can learn about people just by observing their breathing. If you know what to look for, you can practically do a full psychoanalysis! When I start working with new students on their breathing, I can quickly determine whether they hold more anxiety around the future or anger about the past. I can see very clearly what their current emotional state is, and I can tell you whether they're comfortable expressing themselves or if they tend to hold back. The breath betrays what's really going on in the mind and the body, and it never lies.

Imbalances in the breath indicate agitation and dis-ease in the mind. If you start noticing how people breathe, one of the first things you'll see is that we don't inhale fully. For most people, the in-breath is very short, and the out-breath is even shorter. I'm no exception. My breathing was terrible before I learned how to use it. When I walked into Sri Sri's lecture as this uber-skeptical, high-octane lawyer thinking it was ridiculous to learn how to breathe, I could barely inhale for two seconds. There was no elongation. When the instructors taught us the very first breathing technique—an extended inhalation that you hold at the top of the breath and then exhale for a full six counts—I sounded like I was being choked. My throat and my belly were so tight that they were cutting off my breath. I couldn't help it! That's how I was used to breathing all day long while I was at the office, and it continued when I came home at night with my huge folder of case files to review.

I held on to my breath as a way to control and dissociate from the stress I was feeling. My breath would be a little deeper when I was exercising or walking on the beach, which would bring me some relief, but it wouldn't get to the stress I was holding on to in the back of my mind. It couldn't reach all the things I'd swept under the rug in order to function: unresolved trauma from my early childhood, fear of speaking in public, concerns about what other people thought of me, the need to prove myself. But at the end of two and a half days, my state of mind had transformed.

The deeper sources of stress in the base of the iceberg started emptying out of my system.

During the program, I also noticed that my out-breath was full of skips and it would throw itself out very quickly. Most people breathe in with a kind of flutter. It's not a smooth breath in or out. Instead, there are lots of skips in the breath. That flutter is an indication of something going on in the mind that the person is trying to control. It's in the limbic brain, the memories and emotions that are going on behind the very pragmatic, controlled frontal cortex response of *It's cool. I'm okay. Everything's fine. I have it all under control.*

The other extremely common mistake we make is to hold our breath. We hold on in between breaths, and then there's a sudden, short inhale followed by an exhale that shoots the air out. The thrust of the exhale almost makes a "ha!" sound. This tells me so much about a person's mental and emotional state. Last year, I started working with a talented writer, a young woman living in New York City. She had just recently published her first book, and it had received glowing reviews. My immediate sense from meeting her and what I knew of her career was that she was a very creative person, someone who was full of ideas and enthusiasm. To me, creativity means very loose, easy, relaxed, thriving, *free*. But that wasn't what I saw in her breath. When we first sat down together to go through the breathing techniques, I could immediately see how much she held back, how much she stifled herself and her own expression. She didn't really breathe! The reason she came to see me in the first place was because she'd had terrible shortness of breath for years. Her breath was so shallow that it was practically imperceptible, and then, every once in a while, she would inhale very suddenly and thrust out. There were also skips in the exhale because she was having trouble fully releasing the air from her system. I could tell before we even spoke that she was doing the same thing in her mind: holding back her emotions, holding back what she wanted to say, doubting herself and her capabilities. When I told her this, she confided in me that her writing had been very blocked, and we found that it was because her mind was so stuck in the future. Her fear of failure prevented her from being able to just let herself be, and therefore she couldn't let herself really breathe. She was worried that she couldn't live up to her success—that on some level she was not worthy of it—so she held in what she wanted to say.

Through the breath, she started letting go of all the anxiety and self-doubt she was holding on to, and all the buried, self-directed anger that was underneath it. After a few months of doing the breathing, she called me to say that she was writing again. She felt inspired and was enjoying her creative process for the first time in years. Her mind had gotten unstuck from all of her worries about the future, and she could just enjoy the process of exploring her potential. Even if there were some failures along the way, it didn't matter to her anymore because she had regained a sense of confidence in herself.

We hold the breath as a way to put a lid on our thoughts and emotions. The negative past is running the show, and somewhere in the mind, something is stuck. It's stuck in the memory bank, and, therefore, it's stuck in the breath also. Holding the inhale is a way to avoid releasing whatever that stuck thought or emotion is. We are holding out of stress and fear of unleashing whatever deep, dark memories and emotions are lurking beneath the surface of the controlled mind. When I got the call several years ago with the news that my father had passed, I immediately rushed to the airport and bought my ticket right there at the desk. As I sat there waiting for my flight, I started to notice that I was holding my breath. I didn't want to release my emotions because I was in a public place, so my breath was instinctively keeping them contained.

When we hold so much, we eventually start gasping for air. When you're gasping for air, it means there's a lot of emotion that you're reluctant to release in front of others, or, more likely, that you're unwilling to even accept and acknowledge in yourself. So you shove it under the rug by shutting down the breath. It's an artificial clampdown, a way to dissociate and disconnect. The more we disconnect from what we're experiencing internally, the more we gasp for air and then sigh it back out. It's a sign that we're not giving permission and acceptance to our mental and emotional experience.

This isn't something to judge or feel bad about; it's a natural behavior. Of course we don't want to come unglued—nobody wants that! We prefer to "keep it together" rather than go into the deeper levels of what we're experiencing. Instead of using our energy to empty out, which would give us *more* energy, we use so much of our energy against ourselves to keep it all in. If I have a bucket of dirty water, it's going to require a little bit of energy and effort for me to lift it up and pour it out. But to put a lid on the bucket and walk around carrying it will take far more energy, continuous energy, and I will never be free of that load. At a certain point, I've got to lift up that bucket and pour it out.

Now, I'm not suggesting you walk around all day drawing attention to your deepest, darkest emotions. That's certainly not what I mean when I talk about thriving. Instead, it's using some of the breathing practices while sitting, standing, or walking for 5 or 10 minutes to access the deeper things that are going on internally and to empty them out. Then, when you go out into the world, you won't be fighting against yourself by using your energy to hold back your emotions. You'll be more like you were when you were a kid. When something upset you, you had the freedom to express it and let it go. As adults, the breath gives us that freedom to go deeply into whatever we're experiencing and move through it without getting stuck, *and* without needing to express it outwardly.

Clearing the Memory Bank

The incredible thing about the breath is that it's *always* in the present moment. It doesn't go anywhere. It doesn't get stuck like the mind does. Do you see the amazing truth that's hiding here? We can actually use the breath to get the mind out of where it's stuck, to guide it out of the past and future and anchor it back in the now.

Imagine your breath as the string of a kite. The kite flying in the breeze is your mind, and the person on the ground holding the string is your body. All three parts—mind, body, and breath—are interconnected and dependent on one another. Together, they form a single unit. As the string of the kite, the breath is the link between the mind and the body, the bridge between our external and internal worlds. When the winds kick up and the kite starts flying off into the past and future, how do you steady it? You play with the string! Talking to the kite and yelling "Come back here!" when it's flapping all over the place isn't going to work. Instead, you have to adjust the string. You give it more more slack or tighten it up, you add tension to the string, or you jerk it in a certain direction until it hits that sweet spot where it perfectly catches the wind.

If you've ever flown a kite, you know that when the kite is completely centered, the string actually feels like an iron rod. It's no longer loosey-goosey—it's very solid, and the kite is steady and centered. It doesn't move. Even if you let go, it still stays there. This is like the mind in the present moment: solid, powerful, unwavering, anchored in the flow of life. So we play with the string to bring that kite back into the steady flow of the present, and once it's there, the mind operates from a place of calm focus, and this in turn impacts the breath. When the mind is in flow, our breath is as strong as the iron-rod string of the kite.

The breath travels not only on the surface level of the mind but also in the deepest recesses of the mind. It moves through the whole of the iceberg and into the depths of the memory bank, where it can gather and release old toxins—the old thoughts and emotions we don't need to hang on to anymore. The system has to have some life force to go in and release. It's as if you're opening the lid and letting the steam out. When you first start working with the breath, you might notice that a lot of thoughts and emotions are coming to the surface. Bear with it. It's just a sign of mental detox. Let the thoughts surge up or around; don't fight them. If your mind is racing or you're having worse mood swings than a pregnant woman, just invite it in. When we work with the breath, we begin to clear out the memory bank and the emotions that are stored there.

Don't underestimate how powerful and transformative this process can be. Some of the people who have found the most success with these techniques are veterans with post-traumatic stress disorder, who have found a way to confront and ultimately let go of their most deep-seated traumatic memories when nothing else has worked. Tom, a 33-year-old Iraq veteran, was at the end of his rope when he came to breathing as a last-ditch attempt at treatment for his PTSD. Nothing that the VA had given him (handfuls of different pharmaceuticals, several forms of traditional therapies) had done a thing to alleviate the constant anxiety, moral injury, stress, and sleeplessness that he was living with. After several of his friends from the armed forces committed suicide, Tom decided in desperation to walk across the country as a way to try to get out of his own head. Two thousand seven hundred miles later, he realized that what he needed was just to sit in silence with himself.

In three days, he learned the breathing techniques. Tom breathed more deeply than he had in years, and he said that for the first time since he was in combat, he started to *really* exhale. He began to clear out old memories, even the most stuck ones. The experiences were still there with him, but the energetic and emotional charge wasn't so strong anymore. He didn't have to fight to keep the memories buried. For the first time in years, he felt a sense of presence and joy. He recalls walking out of his session, looking up at the gray sky overhead, and thinking that it was one of the most beautiful things he had ever seen. Learning to breathe again allowed Tom to hit the "reset" button on his nervous system. It just proves that the negative past can be taken out of the present and put right back where it belongs: in the past. When that happens, the nervous system can stop reacting to the present and imagined future through the lens of the past trauma. The mind can get unstuck.

We have anecdotal evidence of hundreds of thousands of people around the world and also scientific evidence to back up the benefits of breathwork for PTSD survivors. In a 2010 pilot study, University of Wisconsin–Madison research team studied the effects of Sudarshan Kriya, the stress-relieving yogic breathing practice offered to veterans through Art of Living and the Welcome Home Troops initiative, on a group of Iraq and Afghanistan vets with PTSD.[3] The study, published in the *Journal of Traumatic Stress*, showed that within a week of practicing the breathwork, the veterans already showed lower anxiety, reduced respiration rates (meaning that their breath became deeper and more elongated), and fewer PTSD symptoms. The negative memories of the past lost their power to control the present and future. As Dr. Emma Seppälä, a Stanford University psychologist who worked on the study, explained, "We know that memory is very malleable. What I think is happening is the association between trauma and memory change—they remember what happened, but it's no longer present and now."[4] In simple terms, the emotional charge of the memory is dislodged from the mind, leaving the person feeling present and calm.

Upgrade Your Breathing

The process of relearning to breathe is twofold: (1) discovering the breath as it is, and (2) knowing how to play with the breath just a little bit, which you can do while you're walking or lying down in bed or sitting at home on your cushy sofa. Not only will your breathing be different when you're practicing the exercises, but your breathing in the rest of life will be different too. During a stressful moment, you will suddenly, without any effort, become calmly aware of your thoughts, emotions, breath, and body. Armed with the tool of breath, you can naturally regulate your stress and emotions as they arise. The moment you realize that you're holding the breath, you'll relax, and your breath will elongate again. The by-product of using the breath is a natural state of heightened awareness. This is true mindfulness.

As I've said, the only way to understand the power of the breath is to experience it for yourself. If you're ready to get started, try experimenting with the breathwork exercises included at the end of this chapter. Just dip your toes in, give them a try for a week or two, and notice what shifts in your energy levels and your mind-set.

Breathwork Practices

- **Evening Breath Cycle:** How you enter sleep determines the quality of your sleep. To properly ease yourself into a resting state, try this simple breath exercise: Lie down on your back and place your hands palms down on your belly. Start to breathe normally in and out, holding the breath for a moment at the top of the inhale. Notice the gentle movement of the palm up and down as well as the navel rising and falling. Your palms will begin to feel heavy, awareness will be drawn deeper inward, and you'll start feeling drowsy. Take up to 10 even, rhythmic inhales and exhales, allowing the breath to naturally drop off as you transition into sleep. The moment you feel sleepy, go to sleep. Use this exercise when you wake up during the night to help you get back to sleep.

- **Morning Breath Cycle:** Instead of rolling over and immediately grabbing for your phone when you wake up, start your day by taking a few minutes to breathe. As soon as you wake up, place your hands on your belly again and complete 10 full, deep breath cycles. This quick practice can help you to complete an unfinished sleep cycle and start your day feeling more refreshed and energized. During sleep, the mind processes old stresses and tensions. When you wake up in the middle of a sleep cycle, those old files can stay open, making you feel uneasy, off-center, or agitated. Doing the 10 breaths immediately upon waking acts as a way to complete the stress-processing cycle, effectively "closing down" any open files.

- **Power Breath:** This energizing breathwork practice instantly empties the mind and brings a jolt of energy to the body, and it will literally only take you two minutes. The rhythm is a natural inhalation followed by a short, sharp exhale through the nose. To begin, sit with your elbows bent near the sides of your waist and your hands in loose fists next to your shoulders. As you inhale through the nose, raise your arms above your head and open the hands wide. As you exhale with a forceful thrust, shoot your arms back down with elbows by your waist and bring your hands back into a gentle fist. Repeat for three sets of 15 to 20 breaths for a non-caffeinated jolt to the system. We call this "yogic coffee."

- **Mind-Shift Breath:** We all know about the benefits of taking full breaths, but few people are aware of the benefits of breathing past the full capacity of your breath. Try this powerful "expanded inhalation" anytime you need to shift your mind-set and clear out stuck thoughts. Here's how it works: As you take a deep breath in through your nose, pause briefly when you reach the full capacity of your inhale. After reaching the full capacity of your inhale, take a few more little sips of extra air in. Pause and hold it all in for a moment before releasing fully through the nose. Even two or three repetitions can instantly clear the mind and reenergize the system.

- **Active Acceptance Breath:** As we'll discuss more in Part IV, a mind in resistance consumes a tremendous amount of vital force. When you find yourself fighting or avoiding some situation in your life, close your eyes and notice the symptoms occurring in your mind and body: tightness in the chest or shoulders, shallow breathing, tension in the navel region, racing thoughts, or negative emotions. What you're experiencing are symptoms of stress, the sympathetic ("fight-or-flight") response. Notice all of this, and then take a long breath in as you're feeling these symptoms. Hold the breath for a moment, and then exhale deeply with the sound *hummmm*. Repeat this three times, and your entire physiology will reset itself to a parasympathetic ("rest-and-digest") response. After noticing these physiological changes, go back and repeat the mind-shift breath as described above.

Why humm? That sound that we naturally make so often (think "um-hum") hits right at the center of the head. It's a subtle way to vibrate the hypothalamus and pineal gland, clearing out any negativity.

Again, be your own scientist. Biohack for yourself what these baby steps to breath can do for your energy and outlook. Then decide if you want to explore further.

CHAPTER 8

Meditation
for Busy People

Back in the '60s when mindfulness first made its way to America, it was brought over by teachers who traveled to the Far East and spent months studying in monasteries with Buddhist monks. They learned the practices of the monks, isolated techniques such as concentration and thought monitoring, then secularized and brought those techniques back to America to help people learn to manage their minds. We often forget that the mindfulness practices that are so popular today are actually *monastic* practices. They were designed to be used by monks whose spiritual path required that they withdraw from society and everyday life in order to seek wisdom and divine connection.

You and I are not monks living up in the mountains, waking up at 4 A.M. to meditate for three hours and spending the rest of our days in solitude and silent contemplation. We're just regular people living busy lives, maybe in noisy cities, multitasking and using technology, taking care of our families and careers and bank accounts. While we can borrow these monastic practices and use them to cultivate focus and awareness, it's worth asking ourselves whether these practices designed for monks are what makes the most sense for our lifestyles and goals today.

Vedic meditation (or what I've described as "effortless meditation") was not created for monks. These techniques were designed to be used by "householders," or as the Bhagavad Gita puts it, for "the man of action." They were developed 5,000 years ago in India as a tool to help people like you and me become more engaged in our lives, to be more effective and dynamic in our work, relationships, families, and communities. The practices were less about seeking enlightenment (although they could help you get there too) and more about maximizing energy, vitality, joy, connection, and wisdom—qualities to be enjoyed here in the material world we live in. The goal was not to withdraw from life, but instead to get the most out of life.

Vedic meditation is, and has always been, for people with busy lives and busy minds. It doesn't require you to already have the tranquility and mental discipline of a monk in order to be able to do it, and you don't have to practice hours on end for months and years in order to get anywhere. This is meditation for the active mind, not for the mind that's trained itself into stillness by living in silence and solitude. You don't have to try to get your mind to calm down or stop thinking. What this meditation teaches us is to simply allow the mind to do what it does naturally. There's no trying to control thoughts, no attempts to concentrate, focus, or monitor the mind in any way. In fact, there's no *trying*, period. No effort. As I've said, it's an effortless practice to allow the thoughts and emotions to naturally unwind. The way it does that is by using a vibrational tool called *mantra*.

The purpose of this meditation is to rest the mind, right? It's a break from mental activity. In life, the way our system naturally operates is by cycling back and forth between activity and rest. This is how we are designed: we have circadian rhythms that shift from rest to activity and back again over the course of the day. Based on this awareness, Vedanta divides the day into three cycles of rest: you have eight hours of sleep, and then you also need to add two cycles of meditation during the day to rest the mind. The mind needs rest in order to be vibrant and alive. It needs to be in a state of nothingness to recharge itself.

That's why we call meditation the state of "effortless awareness." When the mind expands and settles down, vital force starts to shoot up naturally, leaving you in the present moment with greater clarity and focus. It's important to recognize that in Vedic meditation, concentration and focus are a result of having *let go* of controlled cognition. The process of meditation itself does not require any mental effort. This meditation is also a way to buy yourself time because it makes the mental faculty more efficient. In addition, when you meditate daily, sleep becomes much deeper, and therefore you need less sleep. That gives you more time to spend in activity. You end up with more time to achieve more in the world.

Vedic meditation is, and has always been, for people with busy lives and busy minds.

Vedanta and Buddhism agree on the fact that meditation is the key to attaining self-mastery. But there are two important secrets of Vedic meditation that make it particularly well suited to the goal of enhancing life and energy. The first is the breath (not focusing on the breath, but the *use* of the breath), and the second is what I call "mind flow," which is the element of effortlessness.

After teaching Vedic meditation to thousands of people, including many practitioners of mindfulness and other forms of meditation, I am compelled to say that the meditation I teach is ideally designed to help us be simultaneously calm and also more active and engaged in life. The self-transcending meditation of the Vedic system is one of the fastest and easiest ways to bring about mental coherence, calm, and dynamism—no matter how busy your mind is to begin with.

Maybe you're wondering, *Can't I just use an app?* Here's why I don't recommend it. The Vedic tradition has treated meditation as part of daily hygiene for thousands of years. It's intended to address the complexity of the human mind; there is a science and a system with years of study, self-observation, and wisdom behind it. It's certainly not something to be casually innovated upon by some tech-savvy person who hasn't a clue what it means to dive deep into his or her own consciousness. I know there are a million "meditation" apps out there that offer convenience; they may offer some surface rest and results, not the full and deep transformative results. There are advantages to that kind of activity, but it's not even a drop in the ocean of what's possible. And on a practical level, it involves more work for lesser reward.

Transcending the Thinking Mind

You already know that mindfulness is not meditation, at least by my standard. So what the hell is meditation, then, if it's not about sitting there trying to focus on your breath? In Sanskrit, the word for meditation is *dhyana*: *dhya* meaning to concentrate, to focus, to localize awareness and attention, and *na* meaning the negation of focus and concentration. It's a state of "no focus" or "no mind." The Vedic word for meditation is the complete opposite of what's been understood as meditation in the West: it's literally a practice of *letting go of focus*.

Let's briefly consider what distinguishes the most commonly practiced forms of meditation. There are a million different ways to meditate, but they all boil down to three broad categories: *focused attention, open monitoring*, and *automatic self-transcending*. The first two categories are the concentration and mental-monitoring practices of mindfulness that we talked about in Chapter 6. Vedic meditation falls into the third category of self-transcending meditation, which is widely known and practiced in the form of Transcendental Meditation. The technique I teach, Sahaj Samadhi, which means "natural, effortless meditation," is also a self-transcending meditation that stems from the same lineage as TM.

Each form of meditation has its own benefits, but the first two categories, by my definition, are not meditation. They're the early stages of regulating attention. As brain-imaging studies clearly show, there's a great deal of mental activity and effort involved. When scientists examined the electrical activity going on in the brain during meditation, they found that focused attention (i.e., mindfulness meditation) triggers brain-wave activity associated with an active frontal cortex, high levels of cognitive control (meaning the controlled thinking processes of the intellect), effortful regulation of attention, and task-oriented thinking.[1] In other words, it triggers the kind of mental activity that we use in our daily lives when we're trying to focus and get things done. It increases the activity of the intellect. A high level of cognitive control is a good thing in the sense that it's a way of "keeping it together"—or, should I say, a way of keeping your "shit under control." Keeping things under control is helpful in certain contexts, but it has the side effect of preventing the flow of new ideas and innovative solutions. If you want insight and fresh inspiration, consider accessing the deeper part of your mind from which your thoughts originate.

Self-transcending meditation has practically the opposite effect of the other two types. It triggers alpha brain waves, which are linked with deep relaxation, creativity, sleep, and very low levels of mental activity.[2] Unlike more regulated forms of meditation, self-transcending practices increase what's called *brain wave coherence*, meaning that there's more unified and synchronized activity across the entire brain. What the practice is doing is essentially creating a more integrated or unified brain, harmonizing every layer of the iceberg from the tip down to the depths of the ocean. In addition, as a direct result of enhanced brain wave coherence and synchronized activity of the entire brain, we also gain the benefit of cognitive control, regulation of attention, and enhanced task-oriented thinking without the hard work or effort of focused-attention and monitoring techniques.[3] This is exactly the meaning of *yoga*. The word literally translates to "integration," "unity," "to 'yoke' together." Our greatest power lies in what the rishis call a "single-pointed," or unified, mind—which is just another way of saying a mind in the present moment.

This is something that can be achieved in a very short period of time, with lasting results—even on your first try. In a study published in 2016 in the prestigious journal *Brain and Cognition*, Dr. Fred Travis demonstrated scientifically that self-transcending meditation truly is an effortless process. The study examined 87 people who had been practicing TM for between one month and five years, testing their brain activity during and after meditation and collecting self-assessment reports. He found that meditators of all experience levels were able to access deep transcendent states. Travis said, "Individuals practicing Transcendental Meditation for just one month reported the same frequency of Transcendental Consciousness experiences during their practice as individuals meditating for five years. This supports the understanding that Transcendental Meditation uses the natural tendency of the mind to transcend—to move from active thinking to deep, inner silence. Extensive practice doesn't make a natural process go any better."[4]

Sahaj Samadhi, like Transcendental Meditation, is an effortless practice, engineered to bring the mind and body into a state of deep, restorative rest. We also call it effortless because the mind naturally wants to move toward the source of joy within. When we allow the thinking process to unwind, it naturally flows back to its true nature, which is the joy, connection, wisdom, creativity, presence, and infinite potential of our consciousness. According to Vedic wisdom, all that we need in life—the creativity, confidence, clarity, all the ingredients for success—we already have. We don't have to do anything special to get it. These things are inside of us; they just get blocked by surface-level thinking. They get covered up by all the judging, labeling, dissecting, and analyzing. So rather than focusing on the surface of the mind, we need to go deeper, down to the very core of our being.

The foundation of Vedanta is the knowledge that who you are, the way you are at your core, is perfect. The quality of who we are innately is *sat*, *chit*, and *ananda*: unchanging, lively awareness and pure bliss. We are made up of these three things. According to Vedanta, if you relax, these three qualities natural-ly come forth. It's the opposite of mental effort. If you take the mind into lesser and lesser effort, your true nature can manifest.

When you relax, these qualities naturally shine forth, as they do in a child.

The way we guide the mind into deeper states of awareness is through the use of a mantra, which is a sound or resonance that has no meaning. The word *mantra* translates to "sound." It's not a word, it's a vibration. Just as a sitar has one sound and a flute has another sound and a piano has another, each mantra has its own sound, and it affects the nervous system in a very specific way. The mantras we use in meditation carry the resonance that we have when we are in our calmest, most peaceful state. We use this vibration as a tool to draw the mind into quieter and quieter states. Effortlessly, the vibration, which functions as a vehicle, takes you beyond the mantra, beyond the process of meditation, and into a state of pure awareness. The mantra is used to "transcend" the process of meditation itself and move into a state of wide-open awareness that is free of thoughts, emotions, and perceptions. We're going into the source of thought itself so that we can change thought, and we're tapping into the source of energy in order to reenergize the entire system. We're letting the mind unwind.

Mind Flow

The beauty of this practice is that it allows the mind to go into a state of nondoing, of total relaxation. It's what I call "mind flow." The mind is naturally unwinding and flowing toward stiller waters. It requires very little of you, aside from the time you take to do it. I love what the musician Moby says of his longtime TM practice: "The thing that makes it effective is you don't have to do all that much. As a profoundly lazy person, I appreciate that."[5] This is the simpler, easier way to meditate. It's relaxing, it's nimble, it conserves energy, and it allows you to sleep better. No one complains that they can't sit through it, and if you do the pre-meditation breathing, you can sit for a long time and it feels as if you've been there only a few moments. You're not struggling to stay in the awareness. You're just naturally observing your inner landscape and allowing the mind to unwind. You're naturally in a state of acceptance. If a negative thought comes, you're not telling yourself, "I'm thinking, I'm thinking, I'm thinking." You just notice that it's there. It doesn't touch you.

> *Like a river flowing back into the ocean, the mind naturally flows back to the still waters of pure consciousness, to the source of energy and intelligence at our core.*

Getting rid of thoughts is not the point. In the Vedic tradition, we accept thoughts as a part of the meditative process. We even welcome them! In trying to resist or label thought, or in trying to meditate at all, we actually end up increasing thought. We're not monitoring or trying to get rid of thoughts, and we don't care if they're positive or negative. We just know that mind does one thing and only knows how to do one thing: think, think, and think. It is the nature of mind to generate thought. Trying to fix or label thought, or judge it, or compartmentalize it, only generates more mental activity. Instead, we are simply floating along the river of thought.

Do you remember those toy monkeys with the cymbals, the ones that wind up with a key at the back? If you think of that key on the back of the monkey as your mind, what you're doing all day long is winding up the key with more and more mental activity. The thinking, analyzing, processing, "right," "wrong," "should be," "should not be"—each one of the tens of thousands of thoughts we have each day is tightening the key. Every single wind builds tension in both the body (the monkey) and the key (the mind). So if you want to release that tension, you have to let go of the key and allow it to unwind on its own. What will happen at first is that the key spins backward like crazy, and the monkey flies all over the place! But that's exactly what we want to happen. You see, when you resist thought, you're resisting the unwinding process and keeping the key locked up tight. You have to know that a part of unwinding is the surge of thought and emotion that comes, takes its time to rise to the surface, and then slows down on its own. Again, the process of meditation is about letting those thoughts and emotions naturally flow toward stillness.

Like a river flowing back into the ocean, the mind naturally flows back to the still waters of pure consciousness, to the source of energy and intelligence at our core. There's so much more life, strength, and stillness deeper in the ocean as opposed to the surface, where the wind is creating lots of waves and agitation. Creativity, enthusiasm, joy, and clarity are much more powerful rising from the bottom of the ocean rather than being generated on the top.

If we're not careful, what we're doing with narrow attention practices is actually putting a lid on the fountain of creativity, insight, and energy that springs up from the bottom of the ocean. Indeed, studies have shown that, while focused-attention meditation improves concentration, focus, and self-regulation, it actually results in *lower* scores on tests of creative thinking.[6] Vedic meditation, on the other hand, has been shown in many experiments to stimulate creative thinking.[7] What you're doing is transcending the thinking mind rather than strengthening and disciplining it. David Lynch, who has practiced TM for over 30 years, describes this beautifully in his book *Catching the Big Fish*:

> If you want to use your full brain, you need to transcend. And then every time you transcend, you carry a little bit more of that transcendental consciousness as you work on your mathematic problems, as you sing, or what have you. Your brain is holding this coherence no matter what you do. It's a holistic experience; it's total brain functioning. And that increasingly becomes a permanent state . . . the more that consciousness grows.[8]

So what is it that's actually happening when you "transcend"? The moment of transcendence is when the iceberg melts into the ocean. It all just becomes flowing water. The common element between the tip of the iceberg and the depths of the ocean is two molecules of hydrogen and one molecule of oxygen. At the moment of transcendence, you let go of all thought, memory, and judgment and arrive at this powerful sense of "I'm here; I am." Sometimes we experience this when we're just moving from sleep into a waking state, when we're half-awake. We don't even know where we are, but we have this clear awareness of *being*. At that moment, we have melted the iceberg. That's transcendence. In that moment, everything restructures itself. When we dip into the ocean, we come back with the power of the ocean, and we begin to melt the ice. Somewhere in the middle of the iceberg, bits of the ice start to soften, and there's a little stream of water flowing back into the ocean. That stream gets bigger and bigger, and then this huge chunk of the iceberg falls into the ocean. The chunk seems like it falls so suddenly, but actually it happened over time as the ice inside was getting softer. The ocean is full of raw life, intelligence, and energy. It's a turbocharge for the system that helps to melt away the blockages that are keeping us stuck. This is what the practice of meditation does for us over time.

At one of my recent trainings, there was a woman who came in to learn meditation as a last resort to deal with her increasingly overwhelming stress levels. This woman was more exhausted than almost anyone I've ever seen. She was a single mother working two jobs, struggling just to make ends meet. She had barely any time for herself, and for the past few months, she also hadn't been sleeping. She complained that her mind was so wound up at night that she couldn't stop thinking and would lie awake for hours. Three minutes into the first meditation with the group, I heard snoring—and I knew exactly where it was coming from! After three minutes of repeating the mantra, she had dropped straight into a deep sleep. The same thing happened in the next three sessions. If I hadn't woken her up after everyone had left, she could have been there for hours. This is what I consider a successful meditation—falling asleep! In our tradition, it's okay to fall asleep during meditation. It's welcomed. Whatever is happening in your internal space, you need to let it happen. This woman's system was operating with a dangerously low battery. Her meter was blinking red. When she was able to quiet her mind enough to drop into that state of transcendence, her body's innate healing intelligence immediately took over. What she needed was rest, and the body gave her a deep, restful state so that she could begin to regenerate herself. *This* is the value of transcendence. We dip into the ocean, and the power of the ocean goes wherever it's needed to serve what is needed.

What's needed, in many cases, is for the mind to confront and release memories that are creating blockages in the subconscious. I recently taught Sahaj Samadhi to a woman who had just lost her son to cancer. Everything you might imagine was going on in her mind: regret, guilt, sadness, grief, anxiety, blaming herself even though there was nothing she could have done. When she first came into my office, she could barely sit still. She'd take a sip of water, then stand up and pace back and forth, then sit back down, then start crying. She told me that there was no way she would be able to sit still for the meditation, but she would try. After the first few moments of her first meditation, tears were rolling down her face, but she was completely still. Forty minutes later, she moved her body for the first time. She opened her eyes and quietly said that she remembered everything from the time when her son was diagnosed with the illness to the moment he passed. Her mind had gone through all the memories that were stored at the water level or deeper in the memory bank. She could see everything, but at the same time, she could see past the pain; the energetic charge had been lifted. After a few sessions, she told me, "I miss my son, but I'm finding a way to sleep at night."

Through this process, the practice can also have a profound impact in relieving depression. An exciting new study published in November 2018 in the highly prestigious *British Journal of Psychiatry* showed that Sahaj Samadhi reduced the relapse rate for depression by more than 300 percent. The study, which spanned five years and included eight research scientists from Western University in Ontario, added meditation to the gold standard of depression treatment: antidepressants and psychotherapy.[9] When we are able to empty the memory bank and let go of the past, we gain the energy that we need to return to the now, experience positive emotions, and take a positive outlook on life.

Preparing the Mind for Meditation

To make the process of meditation even faster and easier, Vedanta strongly suggests starting with the breath. If you are an avid practitioner of Transcendental Meditation, mindfulness, or any other type of meditation, I recommend that you add a few moments of breathwork prior to your current practice. It will change your game, trust me. Instead of spending the first 10 minutes or more of your practice fighting thoughts and internal restlessness, you'll find that the breath clears out the mental clutter in a matter of moments.

Meditation is all about effortlessness, but to make it work in the first place, we have to put in a little bit of effort. Sri Sri compares it to catching a train: "You have to go to the station, buy a ticket, then go to the right platform with your luggage. Once you are on the train, running inside the train with the luggage on your head is not going to make the train go faster." When you sit for meditation, there's nothing to do or accomplish. But before you do nothing, you have to do something.

Again, we're talking about physical effort here, not mental effort. Doing the breathing exercises is no different from doing biceps curls. You just do the repetitions, and then you're done. Whether or not your focus is on the breath, the exercises will shift the nervous system from high alert to rest-and-rejuvenation mode. If you can do a few yoga postures before the breathing to release tension in the body and get your energy channels flowing, that's even better. As Sri Sri explains, "If there is absolutely no activity, then meditation doesn't happen. Yoga and certain breathing techniques take away the restless, jittery energy in you, help you become calm and serene and go deep in meditation." Three minutes of breathing, which requires no focus or concentration, already gives you the ability to sit for an extra 10 or 15 minutes and drop into stillness. Even a shorter meditation will have a much greater impact than sitting there for half an hour with a full mind.

This is why the yogic masters called breathing the "gateway to meditation." It's so much easier to meditate if your system isn't stuck in a hyped-up state of anxiety! What's happening is that, on the level of the intellect, we're telling ourselves that we're relaxing, but in the body and the deeper layers of the mind, the stress and difficult emotions are still there. When you address the stress and open files in the mind *before* you sit down to meditate, your experience of meditation will be easier and more beneficial.

PRACTICES: Unwinding the Mind

Taking some time at least once a day for mental hygiene is a basic requirement for a healthy inner life and high energy levels. We clean the germs and plaque and bacteria out of our mouths twice a day, just as we clean the dust and dirt off our bodies daily. We take off our dirty clothes and change into pajamas at night. But we never think to do the same for our minds. If we want to thrive in life, we have to learn how to shake the dust and debris off of our minds. It doesn't require intense focus or mental effort, but some basic daily upkeep is a necessity. A short, combined practice of breathwork and meditation has been proven over thousands of years to be a highly effective way of doing this.

A book—even this book—can't actually teach you how to meditate. To learn Vedic meditation, some in-person instruction is necessary. (If you're interested, you can sign up for a workshop at an Art of Living or Transcendental Meditation center near you, or head to RajshreePatel.com for more information.)

1. **Flowing Water:** When the mind is stuck in negativity, it means that our energy also is not flowing properly. Our bodies are made up of 70 percent water, and just watching moving water can help us to connect back to that natural movement within ourselves. For this

practice, just sit comfortably by a river or any body of flowing water and gaze at the movement of the water. (An indoor fountain or a video of a river will work too!) You may notice initially that the mind is running its commentaries or getting distracted by lots of thoughts. Just allow the thoughts to come and go. In time, the mind will begin to follow the flow of the water, and the thoughts, emotions, and mental activity will start to drain out. You'll start to shift from mind *full* to mind flow.

2. **Looking Through:** Get the mind flowing with a simple perceptual exercise of looking *to* something without looking *at* it. Simply choose a point in front of you, but instead of looking at it, look through or past it. Keep a soft, defocalized gaze. As you're looking through that point, you will suddenly notice that your field of vision opens up. You're noticing other things to the left or right, above or below. Your attention is still favoring the point, but it's no longer just on that one point. Other elements of the internal environment are also coming into your awareness—sounds or smells or physical sensations. This is a process of letting go of localized attention. Do this for a couple of minutes, and then close your eyes and notice how the mind has slowed down.

3. **Beyond the Horizon:** When you find yourself in a place that has a view into the distance, spend a few moments gazing at the horizon. Initially, the mind is looking—the visual mechanism is engaged—while the intellect is still thinking, thinking, thinking. But if you keep looking at the horizon, then close your eyes, then open and close them again, your mental activity will slow down. Taking in the element of *space* (which Vedanta considers to be one of the five elements, along with earth, air, fire, and water) helps to expand our awareness and shift the nervous system from sympathetic overload to parasympathetic activity.

4. **Hand Gazing:** Hold your hands in front of you, about six inches apart, with your palms facing each other, and gaze gently at the space in the center point between the two palms. You might be aware of what's below or

around the point you're looking at, and then you start to become more aware of your right and left palm. Notice how the awareness is expanding. You went from the center to the side of the hands. Now go past the palms, and simultaneously notice that you're still at the center of the hands. Just be aware of what's in your visual field. As awareness expands to take in more of the space around you, the thinking mechanism slows down.

CHAPTER 9

Living Your Inner Superpowers

I'm a total sucker for Marvel comics and superhero movies (not very "spiritual," I know!). I love when they all come together in *The Avengers*. It's the only movie I've ever gone back to see two days in a row. I think the reason I love these stories so much is because, as fantastical as they are, they really represent human life. Each character—Iron Man, Thor, Hulk, Black Widow, Spiderman—has his or her own unique human weaknesses on the surface, but at the core, they have these superpowers of kindness, courage, commitment, love, compassion, and service. If you look at Iron Man, behind his arrogance is nothing but kindness. Behind the rage of the Hulk is a little boy having a temper tantrum because he can't accept the greed and injustice in the world.

For me, the lesson lies in the recognition that we, like them, also have these superpowers at our core. We are born with these abilities, and we never lose them. They just get covered up by our experiences, traumas, and stories. We are born with the infinite power of everything we need and want to be. It's our birthright. We just need to recognize, connect with, and invite these superpowers consciously into our lives as a daily practice in order to more fully embody the greatness of who we are.

There's a question I love to ask during my talks and workshops. I'll look out at the people sitting in front of me and ask them to raise their hands if they feel that they're operating at their full potential. Ninety-nine percent of the time, not a single hand goes up. It doesn't matter if I'm speaking to a group of veterans or police officers or Fortune 500 executives or students or homemakers. It makes no difference if I'm in India or Brazil or Los Angeles. No matter how much people might have achieved, they don't feel that they have reached their full potential.

You could take this to mean that most people are either self-critical or underperforming, but I don't see it that way. What I see is that all of us have an innate sense of our core Self and the greatness that lies within each of us, the immense potentiality that has not been fully activated and lived. We are able to taste the core of *who we really are*. We know it's there, and we're on an ongoing journey to embody it fully.

We've spent a lot of time talking about the obstacles to our greatness: conditioned thinking, burnout and stress, low energy, and negative emotions of the past and future. But now I want to show you what's on the *other side* of these inner obstacles: we find our greatness, our potential, our true consciousness. It's not something we have to "try" to achieve or become; it's just who we are. We catch glimpses of that radiance when our life force is high and when our minds are at ease, in moments when we're doing something we're passionate about, connecting with the people we love, or feeling a part of the whole of nature and life itself. That greatness isn't just wishful thinking or the voice of your ego. It's something very real. If there is one truth that Vedanta insists on, it's this: you, at your core, are an infinitely happy, powerful being.

The ancient texts tell us that in the same way as we are made up of cells and atoms, we are additionally made up of a substance called "abiding positivity." This substance is known by the name of *satchitananda*, which you know is liveliness (*sat*), pure intelligence of awareness (*chit*), and abiding joy or bliss (*ananda*). It's why we call a newborn baby a "bundle of joy." The dominant substance of the baby is not its weight in physical matter but its pure joy, excitement, and love. All a baby has to do is smile, laugh, or gurgle, and an adult will melt to pieces. What we don't realize is that this quality never gets lost, only covered up. In addition to tools for enhancing our energy and relaxing the mind to allow these qualities to naturally shine forth, the Vedic tradition offers us a set of embodied practices to get there even faster.

> *Just imagine, for a moment, walking around the planet believing that this unlimited power and positivity is who you are! Wouldn't this put a spring in your step and a smile on your face?*

This positive power at our core has many different qualities and takes on many different forms when it's manifested. When we're operating from that place of greatness, we are *resilient* in the face of life's challenges. We speak the truth, and we're honest with others. We behave with kindness and generosity. We're self-aware. We have the disciplined focus to pursue our goals. We maintain a powerful faith in other people and in life itself.

You can think of these qualities that you were born with as your inner superpowers. According to Vedic tradition, these superpowers include kindness, truthfulness, self-discipline, contentment, generosity, resilience, trust, abundance, and more. You can call them "core human values" if you like. They're not emotions or personality traits; they are the substance of which you are made. They are YOU on the deepest possible level. You already know that when you increase your energy levels and relax your mind, you gain greater access to this inner bounty. You're tapping into the very source of your power.

Just imagine, for a moment, walking around the planet believing that this unlimited power and positivity is who you are! You're kind and compassionate, generous, resilient, truthful, happy, self-aware, abundant, mindful, carrying a deep faith in life and your place in it. Wouldn't this put a spring in your step and a smile on your face? It's true! This is who you are; you've just forgotten it. You grew up; you faced challenges, setbacks, and losses; and things started to accumulate in your system. Memories and emotions got stuck in your mind and in the physical tissues of your body. You started to lose touch with that essence you were born with, and you began walking around instead with a head full of narrow beliefs, fixed assumptions about life, and limiting ideas of who you are and what you're capable of. These beliefs and assumptions rolled in like a fog and began to cover up your true nature. The thicker the fog, the more disconnected you felt from your true nature. But just as the sun still shines just as brightly no matter how thick the clouds are, the happiness that is your nature has never lost its radiance. It's just been hidden from your view.

Living Your Essence

Tapping into the source of energy through breathing and effortless meditation—as you've been learning how to do—allows you to naturally and easily return to this core essence of yourself. But there's also a set of daily, embodied behavioral practices that can supercharge the process.

After you've already begun cultivating your *prana*, when you've expanded your mind and awareness through meditation, then the sages say that you can begin to develop these superpowers, which they call *siddhis*. You can also think of them as virtues. You're not introducing anything new or foreign into your system. These things aren't being created in you, they're blossoming in you. This is who you are as your most expanded, vital, vibrant Self. You're simply unfolding those positive qualities that have gotten covered over. Consciously aligning with these qualities that are your nature allows you to blossom into the happiness that you are, the gratitude that you are, the strength that you are, the truthfulness that you are, and so on. What you're doing is aligning your awareness and action with your inner greatness.

We tap into our powers using a series of practices known as the *yama* and *niyama*. If you practice yoga, you've probably heard of them. These principles were outlined in an ancient text called the Yoga Sutras, which were recorded by the sage Patanjali. After describing the physical postures of yoga and the practices of *pranayama* and meditation, Patanjali moves on to the *yama* and *niyama*: active practices of awareness as relates to oneself and active practices of awareness as relates to others. You can also think of them as meditations in action. The *yamas* are practices to improve our awareness of and interactions with others—things like honesty, kindness, and generosity. You practice these things not because it's some kind of moral obligation, but instead because doing so changes the direction of your thoughts and emotions in a way that realigns you with your greater potential. It uplifts your own mind from the very base of the iceberg. It's as much about the way it makes you feel as it is about the way it impacts others. Then we have the *niyamas*, which are the corresponding practices to increase self-awareness and improve your relationship to yourself and your own internal world.

Another way to think of these practices is as a sort of discipline in life, like a code of conduct. If you go on a Vipassana retreat, you have to follow a whole set of rules: you don't sleep on a high bed; you don't write anything down or speak to anyone. You don't follow these rules because someone said so; you follow them because it's what's best for you and your own experience of the retreat. You're refraining from certain actions that lead to mental dysfunction and emotional dysregulation, which ultimately drains your energy and takes you further away from your nature.

The *yama* and *niyama* are not qualities of thought or ways of thinking. Again, they are our core essence. As children, we are kind. We tell the truth without any filters or judgments. We share. We don't steal. We're content with what we have. We get right back up after we fall down. All of these qualities, in the end, are innate to us; we're just tapping into them more consciously. We're not creating another conditioned mind-set that's been constructed based on the past. It's similar to the Buddhist way of practicing compassion. You start out on the surface by using meditations that connect you to your innate sense of empathy. Then you move to sympathetic joy (the practice of finding joy in others' good fortune). Then you move on to practicing loving-kindness, first toward people you know, then toward yourself, then toward all beings. But because compassion isn't a practice—it's your nature—you're just shining light on who you are so the quality can blossom on its own. The practices pave the way for an organic experience of living in accordance with your true nature.

These practices are meant to be *lived*. Remember that the Buddha didn't just meditate when he sat; he was meditative in life. Like the other rishis, Patanjali is trying to help an ordinary householder of his time to live a bigger, better life and to discover his or her own individual height of greatness. That's his objective. He's asking people to do these practices of yoga, breathing, and meditation to raise up their field of energy, and then he says we will naturally live these qualities within the context of our daily activities.

Melting the Iceberg

Again, it's important to understand that these qualities of the *yama* and *niyama* are not of the mind. They're not part of the iceberg at all—they are part of the ocean. Another way to see it is as the hydrogen and the oxygen that make up the iceberg and the ocean. When they're solidified in the form of the iceberg, the qualities get somehow frozen and blocked. What we're doing here is melting the iceberg by aligning the mind with the qualities of consciousness itself. We melt the iceberg by flooding it with the energy and positive qualities of consciousness. It's like an ultrasound machine that breaks down kidney stones so that they can be released through the urine. The frequency and vibration of the *yama* and *niyama* are powerful enough to break down the energetic blockages created by repetitive thought loops and dense negative emotions such as resentment, anger, guilt, blame, and fear.

Instead of using the mind to create change, we're introducing change on the level of speech and action. It's not mental at all! You are simply introducing a powerful intention to shift your speech and action toward a higher frequency and vibration to elevate your state of mind. You don't have to worry about your thoughts at all. You might have aggressive or violent thoughts, you might be dishonest with yourself, or you might indulge in excess internally. That's fine. We start with what we can. Just the awareness of the fact that the thoughts are unproductive brings us back to our innocence. If you're doing the work to keep your energy high, then you will already decrease your vulnerability to these kinds of thoughts. Your thoughts naturally shift to a higher frequency.

Instead of using the mind to create change, we're introducing change on the level of speech and action. You don't have to worry about your thoughts at all.

Patanjali is telling us that another way to tune our thoughts to a higher frequency is by uplifting our speech and actions. To practice kindness in speech, for example, you speak the truth, but in a way that is kind. You don't have to go through a whole thought process about it; you just speak from an awareness of the principle of kindness. Your thoughts will naturally move in the direction of positivity as a result of changing your behavior. Speech, thought, and action are connected, as in the example of the kite. So we play around with our words and actions to change our thoughts. If you become aware of your diet and start eating healthier foods (which is a behavior), you will naturally shift your thinking around food. It's the same idea. The awareness drives the behavior, and then the behavior changes the thoughts, which then reinforces the speech, which drives the action, which then guides the thoughts again in a virtuous circle.

The Yamas: Creating Harmony with Others

What you'll find in the following pages are active practices to apply in your everyday interactions with the people and events of your life. Patanjali asks us to embody these positive qualities in our actions and also to refrain from certain ways of interacting that create disharmony in our relationships and mental dysfunction within ourselves.

You'll find that when you change your behavior, you naturally invite different outcomes in your life. You start attracting different things. Practice these five *yamas* in your daily life, and you will transform your experiences with your family, your co-workers, your friends, and most of all yourself. You can begin by choosing one or two practices, whichever ones you feel most drawn to in this moment, and start incorporating them into your day. When the behavior starts becoming more natural and automatic, play around with adding a second, a third, and so on until you've incorporated all five.

This is not a difficult process. These practices don't require any extra time commitment, just a little awareness on your part. Remember, these are your inner superpowers, and they are available to you anytime you choose to call upon them. Use them wisely and use them often!

1. Ahimsa: Non-Resistance

We begin with the most foundational principle: *ahimsa*, the practice of nonviolence toward all living things. It's obvious that we should refrain from hurting others physically, emotionally, or in any other way. This is a basic requirement of life that you learned when you were in preschool. It's the "golden rule." Not harming or hurting others is the central goal. The other *yamas* all operate in support of this theme. But what if we look a little further into the meaning of *ahimsa*?

In my own interpretation, the deeper wisdom here is that of *non-resistance*. If you think about it, resistance in your relations with others often plays out in acts of disagreement, conflict, and aggression, depending on the intensity of the resistance. Conflicts between warring nations, religious or racial groups, or liberals and conservatives occur on some level because there is resistance toward the other. Our resistance, though not visible or obvious, becomes the seed of hatred and violence.

When you can't accept people as they are, your mind-set quickly becomes "me versus them." You act from a place of fighting, judging, avoiding, or denying that person or group of people, even if it's on the most subtle level. This may never escalate to physical violence, but you can see that there's a certain degree of mental violence there. There's a kind of inner aggression or, at a more extreme state, an attitude of violence. Operating this way hurts us by lowering our own energy and potentiality. When it's externalized, it hurts others too. Resistance on any level makes your relationships effortful. You're working against yourself in order to get what you want. It's an uphill struggle. (We'll explore the mechanics of resistance in greater detail in Chapter 11.)

Resistance toward other people often turns into a resistance to life itself. The living pulse of the universe wants to support us, and what we are essentially doing is fighting or denying that support. Instead of letting the river float us downstream, we're using our energy to swim against the current. As soon as we apply the awareness of *ahimsa* and start to see our resistance in our interactions with others and with life itself, that awareness opens up a channel of energy within us. It creates an immediate shift toward *non-resistance*—meaning a return to the *affirmative state of our natural existence*. We can also call it "active acceptance." When we come into the world, we are totally open, allowing, and willing. We let life come to us. We observe life around us, and then we reach out to do something with it. Fighting against life is a learned behavior that we can unlearn as adults through the practice of *ahimsa*.

Non-resistance can be practiced on three levels: thought, speech, and action. Let's leave thoughts aside for now and look to something more tangible and easier to control. You have control over what you say and do, don't you? It might feel difficult to control your behavior sometimes—for instance, when you're trying to break a bad habit—but for the most part, you hold yourself accountable for your own words and actions. So the practice is to find small ways to align your words and actions with non-resistance. You can choose one single situation each day where you'll refrain from acting in resistance. You might say to yourself, "Today I won't raise my voice at my assistant" or "I'll hold the subway door open for others this morning instead of pushing my way in first." Or you can say to yourself, "My mind has resistance to this." You don't need to do anything, just acknowledge that there is resistance and identify the person or situation.

You can also take a moment at the end of the day to take inventory of times during the day when you were operating in resistance. You're not trying to fix it or tell yourself not to do it, you're just noticing. The awareness in itself changes the way your mind holds on to resistance in the base of the iceberg by introducing this awareness of who you really are, which is non-resistance. When you put your intention on practicing and living with *ahimsa*, even that little bit of attention is much more powerful than anything you do or say. You'll notice very quickly that others meet you with greater openness and acceptance.

2. Satya: Non-Changingness

The second *yama*, *satya*, asks us to examine our relationship to the truth. *Satya* means "truthfulness," but it's also much more than that. On a deeper level, we're talking about a willingness to explore and *be committed to what is unchanging*. Your words and actions reflect a commitment to the highest truth that is available to you in that moment. The principle of *satya* means thought that agrees with words and words that agree with action. To think one thing, to say another thing, and to do a third thing is not *satya*; it is twistedness.

Satya is about walking the talk. If we don't walk the talk, if we're not aligned, we're telling lies or living with them within ourselves, polluting our conscious and subconscious minds. We operate at a lower vibration, and we deflect others without knowing why.

Let's look more deeply at what being truthful really means. If you think about what you consider to be true, at its highest level, it's *something that will always be that way.* It has a permanent and unchanging quality. It's not fleeting, like an opinion or judgment. To practice *satya* in any given situation or interaction, what we do is consider *the most stable point of view.* What's transient in our perception, and what is long-lasting? Again, it's about integrating thought, speech, and action. We are choosing actions that create more than just fleeting results, relying on ideas that are more than fleeting opinions, and looking for long-term instead of short-term gain. One useful technique to try is to ask yourself: *Is my belief about myself or others 100 percent true? Is it true that I'm a failure in life, or am I just experiencing a setback right now?* If you've been telling yourself, "My boss doesn't like me," is this really true, or could there be another reason for his behavior? These kinds of questions can lead us to the more lasting perspective. The most stable and permanent perspective we can have about ourselves and others is exactly what we've been discussing: *I am more than my body, thoughts, opinions, experiences, and emotions. I am made of the energy of life itself.*

When we can keep our awareness on the bigger picture, on what's best for us in the long term, it naturally leads to more stable outcomes. When you practice *satya* in this way, your actions create greater fruit and value. You don't get bogged down in what someone said or did. Your results are enhanced because you are centered, standing on a solid foundation of your commitment to what is, looking at life from a broader perspective. Patanjali says that the practice of *satya* brings peace and the vibration of well-wishes from others. The value of practicing truthfulness, looking with a more lasting point of view, also brings with it the power to fulfill and actualize our intentions.

---

*Ask yourself: Is my belief about myself or others
100 percent true? Is it true that I'm a failure in
life, or am I just experiencing a setback right now?*

---

3. Asteya: Non-Stealing & Abundance

The biblical commandment "thou shalt not steal" is an expression of the basic principle of *asteya*. In the most literal sense, it means "non-stealing." Don't take what doesn't belong to you. Don't steal someone's money or possessions or intellectual property. That's one level of stealing that's obvious, and which we should clearly refrain from, but let's also look to the subtle wisdom beneath the surface.

The real practice of *asteya* is acting from a mind-set of abundance. I'm talking about abundance on a mental and energetic level more than a material one. There's no need to take from others because we already have all that we could possibly need. An awareness of *asteya* means that we catch ourselves when we start thinking, "I wish I had his life," "I'd kill for her job," or "Why am I still alone while everyone else is getting engaged?" Do you see the connection to stealing here? We practice stealing on the mind and heart level far more than we do on the action level. In your thoughts, emotions, and energy, there is a desire to have for yourself what belongs to someone else. When you're operating from a place of competition and comparison—which always stems from a lack mentality—you engage in a subtle form of stealing. There's a part of you that doesn't want the other person to have the promotion, the luxury vacation, the beautiful family . . . whatever it is that you think you deserve but don't yet have.

When you bring your awareness back to abundance, you remember that at your core you lack nothing. Feeling fullness is a matter of realizing that the road carved out for your life is unique to you. No one else can be you. No one can make you bigger or smaller. When you compare yourself or your path to someone else's, you start to become smaller and more disempowered. But when you act from a place of feeling full and complete in your individuality, jealousy, envy, and competition reduce or completely dissolve. You know that the universe will support you and that what is due to you will come to you. There's no need to grab for what belongs to someone else. You can appreciate what others have and what they bring to the table, knowing that their talents and experiences in no way limit your own. Seek out opportunities to collaborate, learn from others, and create an exchange of skills. This encourages a sense of belongingness, and comparison loosens its grip.

Incorporate *asteya* into your daily life by taking inventory of where you're comparing yourself to others, feeling jealous, or wanting what belongs to someone else. Notice when these feelings come up: Is it at work? When you're on Facebook? When you go out for dinner with your more successful friends? Just take stock at the end of the day. As soon as you bring that awareness in, you invite the energy of abundance that is already in you to cut through the comparison.

The next step is to turn that awareness into an opportunity for connection. Sincerely recognize and praise the qualities in the people that you admire, along with their talents and what they've created in their lives. Reach out and see if there are any ways you might be able to collaborate or learn from them. Knowing that you already have enough for yourself, you can generate even more for yourself by honoring and celebrating the abundance of others.

The result of this practice is that it brings more wealth and prosperity into our lives. Patanjali says that this is a direct result of practicing *asteya*: abundance in consciousness brings abundance on all levels.

4. Brahmacharya: Higher Awareness

Brahmacharya is literally translated as "celibacy," but in a modern context, it's usually taken to mean refraining from overindulging in sense pleasures. This may not sound like such a fun idea, but what this *yama* really does is help us conserve our mojo for greater goals. It's about the right use and direction of our energy and intelligence.

We can think of it as self-restraint or self-control, but what Patanjali is talking about on a deeper level is the ability to maintain a broad vision in life. This *yama* is guiding us to walk in the awareness of the highest reality of life. It gives us the ability to direct our energy away from pleasures that seem important in the moment but are ultimately fleeting and costly. Patanjali is moving our center of identity from the body and matter to energy and consciousness. He's asking us to look beyond our immediate desires.

So why do we talk about it in terms of celibacy? It's not some kind of moral judgment about sex being bad. Patanjali is saying that the pursuit of sex purely for our own immediate sensory pleasure can become an obstacle to our greatness. Just look around at the #MeToo movement and all the sex scandals going on at the time I'm writing. The same can be said of any other form of sensory pleasure, whether it's food, alcohol, shopping, TV, or drugs. According to a Vedic understanding of the mind, the senses localize and narrow our attention, life force, and consciousness. They are the wild horses that run the mind. When they're in charge, they shrink who you are. You're no longer in control of yourself. Whatever you want in the moment becomes more important than anything else—and this is a state of craving. At this point, you're operating from a place of very little consciousness. You've lost perspective on the bigness and the scope of your life, your values, and your capabilities.

Narrowed attention restricts our insights, our intuition, and the wisdom to move through obstacles. It moves the mind more and more into fixed positions and creates rigidity of right and wrong. We operate with less heart and with more left-brain conclusions and judgments.

We've been conditioned to see what we want and chase after it, whether it's success or an attractive partner or an ice cream cone, but this behavior limits us. We lose the big picture. We lose our ability to innovate, adapt, and find new solutions to a problem. One of the biggest keys to success is the ability to see from the widest angle possible. Take an example from the world of business: the entrepreneur who holds the widest vision is the most well prepared to execute on his or her ideas.

Practicing *brahmacharya* is not about suppression but about remembering your higher Self. It is the effect, not the cause. Seeing from a wider point of view for a greater goal, you connect to a higher frequency of energy. You're inviting a higher power into your life. This means asking yourself, *What do I need to stop doing in order to create what I truly desire? Will this pleasure lead me to achieving my goal with greater gusto, or is it depleting my energy?* As you will find in a short time of practice, *brahmacharya* brings strength, vitality, and courage.

5. Aparigraha: Non-Possessiveness & Letting Go

We are conditioned in life to always want more, more, more, and to hold on tightly to what we have for fear of losing it. This mind-set is what we are addressing with *aparigraha,* which means "non-possessiveness," "non-accumulation," or as it's sometimes translated, "non-grasping" with the senses. This means *not holding on* at the level of the mind.

We cling to so many things: beliefs and assumptions, grudges, resentments, painful memories, judgments, failures, losses, fixed ideas about the way things should be. The deeper practice of *aparigraha* asks us to stop holding on. Stop grasping. Let go of what we don't need on a physical, emotional, and mental level. This brings a sense of self-reliance and generosity. We know that we have everything we need and more. We know that the universe will *always* provide for our needs, so we don't have to hold on so tightly. We have so much that we can share with others. We can give freely, knowing that what we give will always come back to us in some form. We are free to exercise generosity.

Ask yourself this: What is it in your life that you can't seem to let go of? What is the point of holding on to it? Who is it serving? When you ask these questions, and you're able to just consider the possibility of letting that thing go, you start to free yourself from the negative memories and emotions you're holding on to along with it. Every morning is a new birth, and every night is another death. You get to start your day fresh, with a pure and free mind that is fully in the present moment.

We know that the universe will always provide for our needs, so we don't have to hold on so tightly. We can give freely, knowing that what we give will always come back to us in some form.

In order to create what you want, you have to think, feel, taste, and experience in your own mind a sense that you already have it. This experience can happen only through the practice of generosity. Be willing to share your talents, your gifts, your insights, and your resources. The more you give away, the more you gain and create. The practice of letting go brings clarity about what from your past is holding you back in the present, as well as farsighted vision for your future.

The Niyamas: Cultivating Inner Harmony

Let's turn our focus inward to the *niyamas*, practices designed to bring more awareness to oneself and one's inner life. Whether you start with the *yamas* or *niyamas*, it doesn't matter. They're equally important. Like the *yamas*, the *niyamas* create harmony and vibrancy on all levels of the system. Choose whatever practice resonates with you the most as you're reading, and work on embodying it more in your life, starting with little daily microactions and allowing that awareness to guide your speech and behavior in whatever way feels natural.

You may have heard of an idea used in many 12-step programs called "practice contrary action." If you're not embodying the yama or niyama in your life at this moment, don't worry about it. From time to time, just practice the contrary action to what you would normally do. "Act as if" you are living your super powers. This literally develops new neural pathways and new grooves of habit in your system. Keep a journal. Make a list of small, simple actions and then implement them. Anything to create new grooves. Remember, it's a virtuous cycle and the good will come back to you.

1. Saucha: Cleanliness, Purity & Innocence

Brushing your teeth, bathing, and cleaning your home are basic things that you do on a (hopefully) daily basis. External and internal cleanliness, respectively, are the more literal and the more subtle practices of *saucha*. According to Patanjali, maintaining purity is absolutely crucial for self-harmony.

The way I teach *saucha* includes cleanliness on an internal and energetic level—on the level of your vibe and emotions. If you want to cleanse and purify each level of your system, you need to do more than just brush your teeth and wash your face. You need to have some kind of daily practice to clean your mind and energy field of unwanted clutter and debris.

Cleanliness on a physical level is also rejuvenating for us energetically and mentally. You may not know it, but you're cleansing your mind when you shower in the morning or at night. Water is rejuvenating for every layer of our being; it washes away the dust that's accumulated on the mind over the course of the day or week. You get out of the shower, and you feel refreshed because you've washed something away along with the falling water.

Let's start with our energy hygiene. Showering helps, but we need to do more to take care of our energy. You have to put in some daily effort to keep your vibrations high. You know that everything is energy, so it shouldn't come as a surprise that some level of energetic exchange is happening to you all the time. You are not a solid physical entity; you're a porous being that is constantly exchanging emotions and feelings as energy with everything and everyone around you. The world is full of electromagnetic energetic impulses that you're interacting with and often absorbing into your own system. *Saucha* means being conscious about what kind of energy you're absorbing, which is something you already do naturally. If you have the choice to sit down on the subway next to someone who looks calm and relaxed or someone who's frantically typing away on his or her phone, chances are you'll gravitate toward the first person.

Try bringing a little extra awareness to the energy you're surrounding yourself with, taking measures whenever possible to surround yourself with people, environments, and situations that feel calm or uplifting. Notice when certain people or environments leave you feeling agitated or depleted, and avoid them when possible.

Showers, again, can help to wash off any unwanted energy that you may have picked up. (Cold showers, which stimulate the rising movement of *prana*, are particularly recommended in the Ayurvedic health tradition of India.) If you're out and about, take a little bit of cold water and dab it on the back of your neck for a similar regenerating effect.

The breath is another way to keep energy moving through the system instead of getting stuck. From time to time, when you know you're interacting in a difficult situation, take conscious breaths. Try this technique: When you breathe in, pause your breath at a random moment. When you breathe out, pause your breath again and randomly release. This helps things to not stick to you because when you hold your breath, the mind goes for a moment into a state of suspension. This is something you already do unconsciously. Under stress, we naturally hold the breath as a way to keep ourselves contained and avoid letting anything else in.

When you find that your mind is fixed and is caught up in self-judgment, just ask yourself, If an alien were to see the same situation, what would it say or see?

The other core component of *saucha* is *mental hygiene*. As we've discussed, it's critical to take some time each day to shake the dust off the mind. Even if it's just for five minutes, this is a basic necessity for a healthy inner life. When you practice your daily *sadhana* ("spiritual practice")—a short "time-out" for breathwork and meditation—you're doing important house-keeping for the mind. These practices sweep out the debris that's accumulated over the course of the day. We can clear out the clutter that makes our mind *full* and return to our natural mindfulness.

Finally, on an even deeper level, we can understand *saucha* as a kind of purity and innocence of mind. It's a beginner's mind, the willingness to look from a fresh set of eyes. When you find that your mind is fixed and is caught up in self-judgment, just ask yourself, *If an alien were to see the same situation, what would it say or see?* Be positive and outrageous in your answer. You're aiming here for innocence in the point of view that you hold about yourself. Find the humor in the situation. You're cultivating the willingness to see each moment or interaction as a new, fresh moment untinged by the past. Remember that we are each our own worst critic—we are the hardest on ourselves. Innocence of mind doesn't mean being ignorant or stupid; it means that we're allowing a fresh perspective to unfold through the energy of the universe and its innate intelligence. It brings us to a place of being present in the here and now, using the freedom and unlimited possibilities of the now to create new results. This practice and willingness to invite purity of mind brings greater self-mastery and a more pleasant attitude in life. Sri Sri says it best: "Trust in the innocence of the moment."

2. Santosha: Contentment

The famous expression "Happiness is wanting what you have" is a perfect description of *santosha*, the practice of contentment.

Santosha means being happy, with or without a reason and with or without a cause. It's not the kind of happiness that you think will come some imaginary day when you've gotten everything you want. It's about being content with exactly what you have right now. When you look around at your life, you can find so much to appreciate. If more comes, that's great, but you already have a lot. Patanjali says that if you can find a way to be happy with exactly what you have right now, you cultivate the clarity and mental flexibility necessary to bring even more of what you want into your life.

Santosha stems from an awareness that happiness is our nature. To be clear, there are two different things we're talking about when we talk about happiness. There's outer happiness, and then there's our internal state of happiness. External happiness is fleeting. It's tied to a person, achievement, or possession that we think will bring us fulfillment. We say we'll be happy when we get the new job, but before we can even enjoy the job, we've moved on to worrying about performing well and keeping the job. We can no longer enjoy the accomplishment because our minds have already moved on. This is what the mind does: it moves from one person, object, or event to another. This isn't *santosha*. I'm not discussing this happiness that comes from outside, and I don't think you need my help in finding it.

The second kind of happiness, inner happiness, is what the Vedas call the lasting state of happiness. This is what we're looking for. In this state of happiness, *you* are the source of happiness. Nothing external is needed. When you practice *santosha*, you're tapping into this wellspring of joy and positivity that is completely self-generated.

The practice of *santosha* is simple and immediately uplifting. The next time you become aware that your mind is focused on what's missing in your life, look to see what's there that you can appreciate. If a situation didn't turn out the way you hoped, look to see what you *did* get out of it. It's never all or nothing. There is always growth in failure. There is always love in loss. There is always courage in fear. The real question is: *Can you find it?*

Find some value in whatever situation or interaction you're currently in, and what you'll discover is that this opens the door to a solution or opportunity that can bring greater positivity into your life. Perhaps you were let go from a job, and despite the painful transition, it ultimately provided the fuel that pushed you to fulfill your dream of starting your own business. You're not putting on rose-colored glasses, telling yourself that everything's great and ignoring your true feelings. You're just acting from the awareness that in any given moment there is some positive value in whatever's happening. You're finding gratitude and appreciation for what's here in front of you right now, which brings you to a natural state of contentment.

Being happy with what's right here, right now—which could be as simple as being happy to be alive and breathing—has the direct impact of bringing further happiness and success. Practicing *santosha* is said to bring supreme happiness. The direct gain of this *niyama* is reduced restlessness and a pure, unshakable joy that lights you up from within.

3. Tapas: Self-Discipline & Resilience

Tapas is spoken of in yoga as self-discipline. In my understanding, what Patanjali is really talking about isn't just self-control but also the willingness to lose something in order to gain something greater. It's a kind of resilience and ability to embrace the inevitable losses and hardships that you will face along the journey to realizing your greater potential.

In *tapas*, you practice willingly letting go. It's a kind of conscious self-sacrifice. With *aparigraha*, non-grasping, we spoke about letting go as it relates to others. Here, with *tapas*, we are speaking of letting go or sacrifice as it relates to oneself. Maybe you let go of sleeping in so that you can get to the gym at 6 A.M. because your bigger goal is to be healthier and stronger. You sacrifice financial gain for a year or two in order to make the big career change you've been dreaming of for 10 years. You let go of your mental resistance enough to sit down on the cushion and meditate every day because peace of mind is a priority in your life.

When you practice *tapas,* you're rising above the mind's complaints. Willingly and knowingly embracing a challenge is *tapas.* It builds stamina and creates resilience. When we enter a challenge with a positive state of mind, with conscious awareness, the natural by-product is a surge of life force, along with abilities and skills that you can harness in that moment. This life force is also known as resilience. Nothing sways you; you just go for it with the fullest of gusto. You do whatever needs to be done to reach your larger goal.

It's a phenomenal thing, this *tapas*: consciously choosing to say "I'm giving this up" or "I'm embracing this challenge." We've already talked about how you lose sight of your own bigness when you hold on to something small. The mind narrows, and you lose your resilience and flexibility. To keep your mind wide and cultivate greater resilience, ask yourself each day, *What's one little thing I can give up today?* or *What's the one challenge that I can voluntarily embrace today?* Perhaps it's giving up your second cup of coffee, or dessert, or Facebook, or complaining. Or maybe your challenge is to confront a friend about something he or she did that hurt you, or to take the initiative to lead a big project at work. It doesn't matter how big or small—just choose one thing each day and stick to it.

The resilience of *tapas* also comes from a lived practice of looking back at your life and being able to say, *I've faced so many challenges, but somehow I've always gotten through it.* Even if you thought at the time that you couldn't possibly survive it, somehow you did. Keeping this awareness can help you to better face the next challenge, and the next, and the next.

4. Svadhyaya: Self-Examination & Self-Responsibility

Self-reflection is the work of the fourth *niyama, svadhyaya.* Usually translated as "self-study" or "self-examination," this practice is about stopping to observe your own behavior and ask how you've contributed to a situation or what you might do to improve it. At its core, it's a matter of taking responsibility and holding yourself accountable for your own thoughts, words, actions, and feelings.

It's easy to take responsibility for the things that are going well in your life. It's much more difficult—and much more important—to do this when things aren't going your way.

Svadhyaya tells us: When something isn't working, don't look outside yourself and point fingers at people or circumstances. Observe your own thoughts and emotions, your own inner state. Ask yourself what you could do differently. *What is it in me that needs to change to create the outcome I'm looking for?* This naturally enhances *tapas*, the power of resilience. Ask yourself, *Where does my responsibility lie here?* In the case of a conflict, you're acknowledging that it takes two to tango and holding yourself accountable for your own role. When I get into an argument with one of my brothers or someone I work with, my immediate reaction is to tell myself stories about what the other person did wrong. But *svadhyaya* comes in to guide me to dig a little deeper and reflect on my own role. Often we have a resistance to taking responsibility in new situations. I have a rule that I use in those moments: I tell myself to make up three things that I could have done better or that I can do right now to make a difference. Using this technique is a way to practice *svadhyaya*.

It's easy to take responsibility for the things that are going well in your life. It's much more difficult—and much more important—to do this when things aren't going your way. That's when you really need *svadhyaya*. It's not easy, but it's unbelievably empowering to say, "I created this situation, and I'm responsible for it." Immediately, you stop blaming, you stop being the victim, you stop being stuck, and you start moving forward with your head held high and your mind anchored in the present, with a focus on *what you can do right now.* You move into action.

When you take responsibility for yourself, your own capabilities blossom. You become stronger and more centered. You meet life with acceptance, and life meets you right back with opportunities and guidance. Patanjali says that the result of *svadhyaya* is bringing more divinity into your life. I prefer to think of it as inviting more of the loving support of the universe. All flows to you; you don't have to put so much effort in. Life moves with you and through you.

5. Ishvara Pranidhana: Self-Love & Faith in a Higher Power

The final *niyama, ishvara pranidhana,* asks us to "surrender to the divine." Whether you believe in the divine or not doesn't matter. What Patanjali is talking about in a broader sense is your ability to let go and trust that life will always take care of you. It's your ability to have faith that there is a plan for you. It's another way to grow more trust in yourself. Even during the worst situations, if you can maintain the confidence that there is a bigger plan for you, then you'll remain proactive rather than giving up. Take a look around you: everything in life, the animal kingdom to the plant kingdom to the stars and the planets, is moving in harmony with some order and structure. Why would you be left out of that perfect design?

Vedic wisdom tells us that there is always a greater plan for us, even if we can't see it. When we're lost in the dark and we can't see more than a few feet ahead of us, Patanjali is asking us to connect to the place inside of ourselves that knows that we are always being guided in the right direction. Making the choice to trust in life's guidance and support is what it means to practice *ishvara pranidhana.* It's about being able to say to ourselves, "I know in my heart that I am always moving toward my greater good." I can't tell you how many times I have had to say this to myself the last five years of my life, even after many years of spiritual practice—but that's another story.

There's nothing more powerful than this awareness for boosting your energy, stamina, and outlook on life. If you can live with this kind of faith, nothing can touch you! You find total freedom. You accept and embrace all of your experiences, knowing that they are always there for your own benefit.

When things aren't working out in our lives, when we're struggling and in pain, that's when we need faith the most. Of course, this is also when we have the hardest time finding it. It's so difficult to see beyond the immediate struggles. We had a plan for our lives, and it didn't work out that way—so how can we trust in a bigger plan that we can't possibly see or know right now? When something doesn't work out in life, it is a precious opportunity to practice *ishvara pranidhana*. We can do this by stopping and asking ourselves to reexamine our present failure or loss in the context of the whole journey of our lives.

Think about it this way: When you're on a plane, and it's taxiing on the ground, you can hardly see anything. You have to wait until the plane is at cruising altitude before you can get that broader view of everything around you. When you're up at 35,000 feet, you can see so many possibilities from that broad perspective. You see that there aren't just one or two roads that lead to Rome, there are many. There were always a thousand different ways to reach the same place in your life. *Ishvara pranidhana* is about letting go of your righteousness and your fixed positions about "the way things should be." Maybe the relationship you wanted didn't work out. Maybe your business or your marriage failed. You didn't get the job. You lost a loved one. You got an unexpected cancer diagnosis. When life isn't going the way you planned, you can say to yourself, *It's true that I feel like hell is freezing over right now, but I trust that there's a larger plan, even if I can't see it.* In moments of hardship, loss, failure, and disappointment, if you can trust in the benevolence of life, you will find peace. You'll find the energy and mental strength to deal with the unexpected and forge a new path for yourself. It's in this state of surrender that we actually move through the pain of the difficult moments of our lives instead of tucking them away or avoiding them. Seemingly ironically, it's in a state of surrender that we are being truly courageous by choosing not to run away.

What we're doing is coming to trust in a *loving force* at play in our lives. At its deepest, this practice is about love and connection: love for oneself, love for family and friends, and love that expands to include all beings. It's a love that excludes no one, least of all ourselves. Love that is our own nature and the nature of life itself. This is where you move into a sense of connection with a higher power or, if you don't believe in a higher power, a sense of connection to the whole of life.

Remember your journey is from the outside in as well as inside out. The more vital force you have, the more you will naturally live your life from your superpowers—and the more you express your superpowers, the more life force you will have available to you.

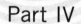

Part IV

UPGRADE YOUR OPERATING SYSTEM

CHAPTER 10

Mastering Your Mind-Set

If I asked you what your mind-set is right now, what would you say? Is it positive or negative? Optimistic or pessimistic? Fixed or open-minded? When I use the word *mind-set*, I'm referring to the quality of the state of mind from which you think, act, and feel. We tend to think that we operate from many different mind-sets in our daily life. We assume that there are a number of lenses through which we perceive, think, feel, and believe. But according to Vedanta, the mind has only two basic modes: we are either operating in resistance, or we're operating in craving. The energy of repulsion or the energy of attraction. We're either pushing something away or pulling something toward ourselves.

Through keen observation and self-study, the rishis discovered again and again that our perception has only these two possibilities. When the intellect processes all the information coming in through our five senses, it distills it into one of these two possible points of view, which the Vedic tradition calls *raga* (attraction) and *dwesha* (aversion). We're either chasing after something, or we're running away from it. We want it, or we don't want it. We like it, or we don't like it. It should be, or it should not be. For everything we experience in life, there is a response of either attraction or repulsion. Very rarely do we perceive from a neutral point of view. When we're at neutral, we're simply in the present moment, observing without judgment.

Being at neutral is not a problem. It's resistance and craving that are the problem. I know it's difficult to wrap your head around, but these two mind-sets are the only things that make us miserable in life. If only we could recognize this push and pull as the cause of the limitations we feel! When we're in resistance, we're miserable. When we're in craving, we're also miserable. But we don't see it. Instead, we point our fingers at a million different people, objects, and situations that we think are the cause of our unhappiness. Today it's our job, and tomorrow it's a headache. The next day it's a credit card bill or an unpleasant conversation. We point to the changing objects of the external world and say, "That's the problem," but this is nothing more than the mind's stories.

Getting stuck in this endless push-pull not only drains our energy but also gets us even more trapped in the cycle of past and future. Because a mind in resistance and craving is never at ease, our stress response stays locked in the "on" position. The deeper the groove of these mind-sets, the more rigid, contracted, and closed our minds and our lives become.

Pick Your Poison

For each person, one mind-set is more dominant than the other. Some of us move in life propelled by the force of attraction, while others move repelled by the force of resistance. We each pick our own poison. Either way, at some point, one leads to the other. Unless we can stay in a state of high energy and awareness, we spend our lives swinging in this pendulum of attraction and avoidance.

It's not always easy to recognize when your mind has veered off-center. I'll give you an example from my own life. When I first stumbled upon these Vedic teachings, it was completely unexpected and eye-opening for me. I discovered this whole new world of possibilities. Suddenly, I couldn't believe that in all my years of education—from primary school to law school—nobody had taught me to look inside my own mind. Once I saw the value of that, all I wanted was to share it with others so that they could find the same benefit that I had. I had such a clear vision of what these teachings could do for humanity, so I dove into the work headfirst with the full force of my passion and commitment.

And let me tell you, I went *full on*. I applied the same ambition and drive I used to make it through law school and become a successful prosecutor in Los Angeles. I focused all of my energy and internal resources on spreading these ancient practices that I'd come to believe in so deeply. We taught hundreds of thousands of people in 35 different countries within a period of just a few years.

But I didn't realize that the fervor with which I dove into the work reflected a mind-set that can be categorized, on some level, as craving. I was working long hours, I was constantly traveling all over the world, and I started to lose my basic sense of time and space in the process. I was all activity and not enough rest, working 18 to 20 hours a day to get this message out to people. While I kept up with my daily breathwork and meditation, the number of hours I was putting into activity were not in balance with the hours of rest. It was exciting and fulfilling work, yes. Nevertheless, there was an imbalance in taking care of my health and taking time for myself and my relationships.

There's nothing wrong with having, wanting, and achieving—but when you get so caught up that it becomes the center of your identity, then it limits the field of possibilities that you're operating and creating from.

For all the time I'd spent studying and learning to manage my own mind, I still found myself slipping back into old, conditioned mind-sets. As a child of Indian parents, as an immigrant, and as a lawyer, I was hardwired to strive for achievement and success at any cost. Ultimately, I realized I had to pause and re-center myself to avoid a burnout. The lesson here is that the reasons are irrelevant because we're still operating from mind-sets that are destructive to us.

These mind-sets are often difficult to recognize because they're so tied up with the things we care about most in life. They're intertwined with our deepest dreams and aspirations. You resist your child's health diagnosis because your family is the most important thing in the world to you, and you want nothing more than for them to be well. You have an intense craving to quit your job and travel the world because you deeply value freedom. You become feverish about making an impact with your creative venture because you genuinely believe it can change the world.

This isn't something to feel bad about. The Bhagavad Gita says, "Attraction and aversion of the senses to their corresponding sense objects is unavoidable," meaning the mind is wired this way. It's part of our basic operating system. But the Gita also says that when these mind-sets control us, they become an obstacle to our greatness. When left unchecked, when unconscious, they cause problems in our lives. When we get stuck in what we want or don't want, we lose our greater potentiality. We are bigger than our wants, our achievements, and our goals. There's nothing wrong with having, wanting, and achieving— but when you get so caught up that it becomes the center of your identity, then it limits the field of possibilities that you're operating and creating from. It takes you further away from the positive qualities at your core and reduces your ability to accomplish what you want.

We know that the essence of who we are is joy, love, connection, and vibrancy. Ironically, this is also the reason we start operating in resistance and craving to begin with. We're seeking to return to our greatness. We're trying to get back to our nature. The problem is that we become confused about how to get there. We think that in order to find joy, we need to chase happiness and run away from pain and failure. It's an exhausting journey that only takes us farther away from our potential.

Examining Your Operating System

What I'm asking you to do now is the work of deep self-reflection. Once you're able to see how these mind-sets are driving your thoughts, your behavior, and your life, you won't be able to *unsee* it. It's a rude awakening, trust me. If you can identify your mind's basic tendencies, you become very conscious of what's driving your thoughts, words, and actions. When resistance starts kicking in, you'll be able to identify what is driving you at any given moment. There's great value to this soul-searching because when we become aware, we automatically rise above. Our mind-set expands, perception becomes pure, and expression becomes clear. That's where change begins.

As with a computer, we're looking at the operating system. Is it a PC or a Mac? Is it DOS or Linux? What is it that causes the computer to crash? What programs are draining the most battery power? Once we know how we operate, then our perception starts to shift on its own. By itself, the ability to recognize the mind's tendencies lifts our energy. We start moving out of autopilot, the submerged part of the iceberg, and acting from a more conscious place. We're not using more mind to solve the mind's problems. We are becoming more *aware*. Awareness is not thinking; it's a deep knowing with the power to redirect the mind at all levels.

The moment we become aware of how we're operating, the mind instantly expands. The mind that has become negative, tight, and pinched suddenly opens up, and our perspective widens. It comes back to center, to a place of neutrality, to the present moment. Awareness invites more energy and gives us the motivation to enhance our energy further. With that, let's look more closely at these two core mind-sets and the effect they're having on our energy and our lives.

CHAPTER 11

From Fighting to Flowing

Being a writer is a very new experience for me. For years, I've resisted the idea of writing anything, let alone a book. People have been telling me for decades to write, but I never wanted to. Sri Sri always said that there was a book inside of me wanting to come out, and I just kept telling myself and everyone else, *No, no, no, I don't want to write a book.* Who wants to sit in a cave with a computer and a cup of coffee? I like to connect with people, share, talk, and express ideas with an exchange of energy. Writing to me always seemed isolating, with very little human engagement.

But eventually I decided to follow Sri Sri's lead and gave in to the idea of writing a book. So I did what any aspiring author would do: I gathered my thoughts, created a proposal, and found a publisher. I began collecting all these teachings from my lifetime of work and putting them down on the page.

Immediately after I began on the book, my resistance to writing came back to rear its ugly head. *No, no, no, I don't want to write a book.* I hate writing! It's just not the way my brain works. Even as a lawyer, I managed to get by writing as little as possible. I managed to silence that voice enough to get on with the work, but it still wasn't gone.

There was some level of resistance in my submerged mind, and it started manifesting itself in all kinds of crazy ways. My computer broke down not once but twice. I developed a serious eye infection that persisted on and off for the entire duration of the writing process, often making it impossible for me to look at a screen. Because of a digestive problem, I ended up on a heavy course of antibiotics that clouded my thinking and zapped my energy. My house had not one, not two, but three major water leaks, forcing me into a hotel and eventually out of my home for one full year. And these are just the highlights! Even while I was actively writing, on a subconscious level, my mind was still saying no. Internally, I was pushing the opportunity that life had given me away, and life responded by making it more difficult for me to write. It's not so surprising when you think about it. This is what resistance does: it makes things more difficult. When you're at a cycling class and you want to make your muscles work harder, you add *resistance* to the bike. Your legs then have to pump harder to go the same distance. When you add resistance, you create a tension that forces the muscles to exert more effort.

What Vedanta teaches, and I firmly believe, is that there are no accidents in life. What's happening in our lives out there in the world is an expression of what's going on in here. My internal "no" was manifesting in external situations that created greater struggle, difficulty, and negativity. At a certain point midway through the process, while I was lying in a hotel bed with a pink, swollen eye and a crashed laptop, squinting to read off a printed-out chapter, I just started laughing. And once I started, I couldn't stop. The universe has such a sense of humor sometimes! I said to life, "Okay, you win! I accept all this craziness; I accept the challenges of this writing process; I surrender." And once I accepted the struggles, they began to evaporate. The writing began to flow more easily, and the path ahead of me became more clear. Once I shifted the gears of my mind, the uphill climb became a smoother ride. There were still bumps in the road, but I was no longer fighting against them. I simply accepted the challenges and did what I had to do in the moment to deal with them.

So what is this thing called *resistance*, really, and how does it mess so much with our lives? Simply put, resistance is the *conscious or unconscious unwillingness or refusal to allow anything in*. We can also call it non-acceptance, aversion, or avoidance of what is. It's all the same thing. We don't like something, so we push it away, pretend it's not there, get annoyed or angry about it, throw punches at it, or shove it under the rug. For the most part, resistance is our default mind-set in life. We do not, and we feel we cannot, accept our lives as they are. You should know enough about energy by now to immediately be able to see that resistance is an extremely energy-inefficient mind-set. It creates stress throughout the system and gets us more stuck in the past-future cycle. If we want to upgrade our energy and our lives, addressing the mind's tendency toward resistance is a crucial part of the process.

Becoming a Good Energy Conductor

Resistance is a force as real as gravity. It creates tension and contraction in the mind in the same way that adding resistance in a workout creates contraction in the muscles. We can understand what resistance does to our energy by looking at it from a simple physics perspective. Think back to that high school science class where you learned about how electricity works. You were taught that electricity is basically the movement of electrons and that any object that's powered by electricity harnesses the flow of electrons as its energy source. In physics, the rate at which an electrical charge flows through a material is called a *current. Resistance* is the term used to describe a material's *tendency to resist the current.* When the current is moving through a narrow pipe, for instance, there is more resistance than when the same current is moving through a wider pipe at the same pressure. It makes sense, doesn't it? You know that everything in life is energy. We human beings are just more complicated conductors of this electrical energy that we call life force. That's essentially the function of the brain and nervous system: to send and receive electrical impulses or, in other words, to be a *conductor* of electricity. In physics, a good conductor of electricity is one that has a low degree of resistance, and a poor conductor is one that has high resistance. Unless you are somehow magically able to defy the laws of physics, you work exactly the same way.

Your mind—and the physical brain that gives life to your mind—is a good conductor of energy when it has a low degree of resistance! A narrow, pinched mind creates resistance to the flow of energy. It's a poor conductor. When there's more resistance, the energy is not able to flow properly. It's that simple. But when your mind-set is wide open—fully in the present moment, with acceptance of what is—energy can flow freely through you, and you can harness that energy to manifest your own goals and dreams.

If you truly realize how your mind is stuck in the past and the future and functioning from a state of resistance, you will have a reckoning moment of Holy shit, what am I doing to myself?

Please slow yourself down right now and really look inward and hear what I'm saying. Resistance is a mental phenomenon that is a force like gravity. It has the power to restrict the free movement of our life force. You can interpret *life force* to mean your heart. Remember, life force is not some mechanical, inanimate electrical energy; it is your heart quality. It expresses itself in movement but also in qualities such as love, compassion, kindness, connection, intimacy, care, service, and so on. Life force also operates all your cognitive functions. When your mind goes into resistance, you start to become more rigid in the use of your mental faculties. To make matters worse, you put a wall around your heart and its expression. The degree of resistance determines the size of the wall and the level of rigidity and control. It stops you from letting life and love come in.

Being a good conductor of energy is what we've been talking about from page 1 of this book! To harness the energy of life within and around you, the mind must be wide open. When your mind is stuck in resistance, you are literally opposing the flow of life. Vedanta speaks about resistance and what it does to the system. In resistance, the subtle energy channels contract (and if you don't believe in energy channels, think of it in terms of your nerves, your veins, and your arteries). Everything tightens and narrows. Your mind becomes a tight, contracted, narrow pipe, and the energy of life can't flow through it. When this happens, we become drained and depleted, rigid and fixed. As the battery drains, the mind narrows further, and we feel more and more disconnected from others and from life itself. We are literally cutting ourselves off from the source energy that nourishes us.

Awareness is a necessary first step to breaking free from this toxic mind-set. If you truly realize how your mind is stuck in the past and the future and functioning from a state of resistance, you will have a reckoning moment of *Holy shit, what am I doing to myself?* It's a wake-up call. That revelation in itself becomes the tool you need to break free.

Reexamining Resistance

You'll see that people who live in resistance become hardened to life. Notice this in your friends, your family, and your coworkers. That person who is always complaining and fighting against life—how does he look to you? If you're paying attention, you can see it in these people's faces, in their eyes, in the way they carry themselves. The resistance has worn them down over time, not just mentally but also physically. These are the people who are often very tired at the end of the day and need to sleep for many hours to recover. People who have operated from resistance for many years are tough, closed-off people. They don't allow anything to penetrate them. But I'm not just talking about a certain kind of person; I'm talking about everyone at one time or another. We all operate in resistance in at least one area of our lives.

This comes up in every single course I teach. There is always someone (and sometimes a number of people) functioning from a place of massive resistance and completely unaware of it. They wonder why things aren't working in their lives, why everything is such a struggle, why there's no support, why they can't find the partner they want or the job they want. It's no mystery to me what's going on. Resistance creates contraction and negative emotions, which creates a perception of struggle, which manifests externally in actual struggle. The person is unwittingly pushing away the opportunities that they want because they can't accept what's right in front of them. It's a predictable chain of events.

For the sake of your energy and your life, you must shift your mind-set from resistance to the opposite of resistance: non-resistance or *acceptance*. The moment you entertain the possibility of acceptance, your mind expands. You are flooded with energy. The moment you stop narrowing in on an issue and can begin to see things from a broader point of view—being able to say, "It's okay; everything is going to work out just fine"—you increase and stimulate the flow of life force in your system.

If I'm dealing with some challenge, and I contract my mind, my point of view becomes one of resistance: "Wow, this isn't the way it's supposed to be," "This isn't going to work out," "I don't want to deal with this again," "This is a serious problem." The narrower you become, the more quickly you drain the battery with negative thinking and emotions. You lose the ability to be clear and process things neutrally. You lose the ability to feel joy and excitement. But the moment you say, "Oh well, that happened. I'll make it," the energy starts flowing again. It's like taking a big inhale after you've been holding your breath. When the mind is in acceptance, life force shoots up. Mind in other states sucks life force. There's a constant manipulation and calculation and strategizing that goes on, which is just a form of resistance.

But the moment we're in acceptance, we recenter and simply say to ourselves, *This is how the situation is. This is what I need to do to fix it.*

As I mentioned, my house was flooded while I was writing this book. When my husband called to tell me what had happened, I immediately said, "Wow, that means that we're going to get to design a new kitchen." That was my knee-jerk response. A few friends of mine who were sitting next to me when I got the call were completely shocked. For two days, they kept coming to me to say how sorry they were about the flooding and how terrible and inconvenient it was. But I had vibrancy and vitality because my point of view, my mindset, expanded from a place of acceptance. My friends' minds contracted. They lost energy while I gained energy from the same situation.

Saying No to Life

What we're talking about in this book is how to conserve and enhance the life that we were born with. Resistance is an absolutely critical part of this conversation because it's one of the major internal forces that takes our own life away from us. It leaves us dull, drained, lifeless, bitter, struggling. It is literally a slow death. We pay a price for operating in resistance, and that price is our lives.

The Vedic tradition says that in resistance, you are not allowing life's possibilities to come to you. You're becoming a stone wall as opposed to a porous net. The expression of heart qualities in your life shrinks as your mind operates in resistance. In resistance, intellect functions with strong judgment, persistence, and stubbornness, and the heart lags behind. You live more from your head than from your heart.

Here's another physics analogy to help you understand what's going on energetically when your mind is in resistance: Imagine that someone is pushing at your door from the outside. This person is applying 100 units of force to try to push down the door. You're there on the other side, and you really don't want that door opened! You don't want to let that person into your space. So, to keep the person out, you have to apply 100 units of force in order to create enough resistance to keep the door shut.

It takes much more energy to keep things out of your own head, your internal house, than it does to just open the door and invite them in. Instead of using 100 units of energy to resist the person, you could use 30 or 40 units of energy, maybe 50, to speak to the person and deal with whatever it is. Let's look at a real example. Sometimes we have to shut our doors to people or situations in our lives—a family member, a friend, an ex-partner, or a job. If there is no emotional charge in your system about the person or situation, then it's as if you opened the door, said thank you and good-bye to the visitor, and moved on. If, however, you find yourself trying to avoid the person, if you get charged up when the person's name comes up or you feel upset when you have to deal with the person, then know you are using your own energy against yourself. This is an indication that your mind is in resistance. It means you are draining a lot of your potential, effort, and energy in order to keep the person or the situation under the rug. You have not opened the door and dealt with whatever it is. You have not moved on.

Within yourself, too, keeping your emotions at bay requires so much more energy than opening the door and just allowing them to move through. You think it will be easier and more efficient to try to avoid life's challenges when really it saves much more time and energy to just open the door, welcome the challenges (and the opportunities) in, and find a way to deal with whatever is there. You can't control what shows up at your door, but you do have control over how you greet it. If you could see that the nature of life is change, that everything is short-lived and impermanent, you might realize that there's no point in using your precious life force to push away what life brings you.

*What you resist persists, and what you accept
flows. When you invite life in instead of
pushing it away, your life starts to work
for you rather than against you.*

What if you took that same 100 units of energy that you're using to keep the door closed and used just 50 percent of it to go after something you want? What if you used it to risk happiness, to risk success, and to risk pursuing your dreams? You would completely change the dynamics of your life. Your outlook would be transformed. You'd make different choices. The way you relate to the people around you would be completely changed. Instead of walking into the office feeling resentful for having to be there, with your shoulders tense and stomach tied into a knot, distracting yourself by wondering when you'll finally find a new job, you would feel so much more laid back. That doesn't mean you'd be careless in what you're doing or ignore your true feelings about a situation; it just means that you wouldn't be trying to protect yourself from experiencing the basic reality of the situation. You wouldn't be trying to push it away. Instead of looking for ways to avoid risk and failure, you'd look for opportunity. You'd be able to skillfully avert challenges and resolve them when they arise instead of wasting your energy scanning for potential problems before they even happen. As I've said, where our mind goes, that's what follows in our lives. When you assume and anticipate problems, well, problems have a way of finding you.

Just imagine the energy it takes to walk into your office with your body contracted in resistance versus walking in and accepting the way things are—including accepting the fact that you don't feel great at your current job. Instead of staying narrow and closed down, you'd become that wide-open pipe, just allowing the experience as it is to flow through. You'd find things to enjoy in your day, and maybe you'd take on a new project that you'd enjoy or make friends with a new colleague.

You might even start to invite new opportunities in. Isn't it funny how, when you finally accept the job you hate, a new offer pops into your inbox? That's always how it works. And then another opportunity comes after that one—when it rains, it pours, as they say. What you resist persists, and what you accept flows. When you invite life in instead of pushing it away, your life starts to work *for* you rather than against you. Remember, this energy of life wants to support and uplift you: when you take one step toward acceptance and trust, it goes 10 steps further in supporting your thriving.

What Are You Committed To?

If you're thinking that this doesn't apply to you, I invite you to dig a little deeper. I guarantee you that there is at least one area of your life in which you are operating in total non-acceptance, avoidance, and aversion, and it is draining your energy tremendously. You're just not aware of it. The tricky thing about resistance is that it often operates on an unconscious level.

There's a simple question I use to help people determine if they're operating from a mind-set of resistance or one of acceptance: Are you committed to making sure that you're happy in your life, or are you committed to making sure you're *not unhappy*? Are you committed to living a life that you love, or are you committed to avoiding a life that you don't love? The way you answer this question tells me everything I need to know about your mind-set and how your life is going. If you're committed to being happy and loving your life, then you will be thriving. If you're committed to avoiding unhappiness, then you'll have a lukewarm life.

But the answer isn't always as obvious as it initially seems. I've posed this question to thousands of people, and inevitably 90 percent or more of the room will raise their hands to say that they're committed to being happy. Then I'll prod them to look deeper: Are you so sure about that? Imagine that you're sitting here, and there's value you're gaining in this talk, but the person sitting in front of you is too tall and you can't see. What do you do? Do you sit there and take in the value that's present? Or is your mind stuck in *This guy is too tall and he keeps moving and I'm not getting as much out of this workshop as I wanted to*? Well, I'm sorry to say that this is resistance. You're operating to make sure that you're not uncomfortable. Do you see that your effort, attention, and energy are spent not on making the most of your experience but instead on trying to minimize your discomfort? You want to cut his head off. We don't risk being happy. If we did, we would sit back, relax, and find the happiness and value in any situation—or calmly move to another seat. But we don't do that. Instead, we fight against the airport delay, the minor inconvenience, the bigger setbacks and failures, the inevitable challenges in life.

Do you really believe that you're operating to be happy, vibrant, achieving, completely in the flow of life? This might be what you say you want, but in reality your mind is operating from the second option: you're here to survive, to get by as best you can, to try to make sure some shit doesn't happen. It's a very different principle. The first option is acceptance, and the second is resistance. When you are committed to being happy, you're naturally more accepting, allowing, and open to new ideas and directions. It's when you're committed to avoiding pain and unhappiness that you can't accept your life as it is.

Resistance is fear-based operating. It's fear-based choice making. What you're negatively focused on is what you create more of. If your focus is unconscious, it's even more powerful. Something that you're keeping a secret, whether it's an exciting or a damaging secret, bubbles with energy inside of you. It has more power in you than something that's out in the open. What if someone finds out? It eats away at you; it keeps you from being able to sleep; it drains your life force. It takes more energy because it's happening under the rug and you have to devote your internal resources to keeping it suppressed.

Think back to the journey of past and future. The moment the mind goes into resistance, we start on this journey—*shoulda, woulda, coulda*. Why is it that you want to shut the door and keep out whatever's on the other side? It's because of a nega-tive anticipation of the future that's based on something that happened in the past. There's fear because you're carrying these old experiences into your present and future. You've been hurt, rejected, disappointed in the past, so you use all of your energy to push against that door to make damn sure it doesn't happen again. *It didn't work out for my mother, it didn't work out with my business, my last relationship didn't work out, I guess I'm just the kind of person that things don't work out for.* This kind of thinking is an aggravation of the frontal cortex: it's the intellect using its own power against itself. On every level, we're burning out our system. The intellect overthinks, and the memory bank goes into defense mode to try to protect us from future pain. The limbic brain starts feeding negative memories up to the frontal cortex, which fuels the resistance even more. More thoughts are generated. Clarity of mind is diluted, confidence is shaken, op-portunities are lost. Here's where it comes back again to karma, our bondage to the past: *you end up inviting in the very same result that you've been trying to avoid.* You re-create the same past situa-tion that's making you so afraid in the first place.

Excuse my language, but as you can see, resistance is biting and pinching us in the ass. That's because we know intuitively that who we are innately—our larger potential and greatness—is far bigger than the limitations we find ourselves living within. No wonder it pinches! We're trying to get by, preserve what we have, avoid discomfort or getting into trouble. We're telling ourselves on repeat, *I don't want to do this* and *I don't want that to happen.* But because we're not living up to who we know we can be, we feel the pinch—from the inside, like a slow cancer destroying the system. Or a leaking battery draining the whole machine.

The True Cost of Non-Acceptance

Most of the people I meet and work with are so stuck in resistance that their lives are now about just trying to get by without things falling apart. They don't risk anymore; they don't go for it. The notion of "going for it," in itself, means letting go of resistance. It means that you stop holding back and you dive in headfirst—or should I say heart first? As a leader, as a partner in love or business, no matter what role you're in, that resistance is what makes you feel tired, stuck, and incapable. It's what keeps you on the sidelines of life rather than out there in the arena. You wear it like an armor to protect yourself from the negative future that you fear. Instead of using the energy to explode out and create more, you're using the energy against yourself to hold back. Your own life force is being internalized and used against you.

Close your eyes for a moment and think of a situation, person, or place that you can't accept. Bring the details to mind: the person's face, what the person looked like in that moment, the environment you were in, how you felt. Now bring your awareness back to yourself. What do you notice? Maybe your heart rate goes up, body temperature rises, breathing becomes shorter and tighter, negative thoughts and emotions bubble up. Notice how non-acceptance impacts the *whole system*. It sends a signal to every faculty to go into stress response: fight, flight, or freeze. It doesn't matter whether the situation is happening to you in that moment or not; the mind in stress responds the same. If you're sitting in the peaceful mountains and I ask you to think of something you're stressed about, you'll no longer be in the peaceful mountains; you'll be sitting in traffic on the 405. Every parameter of success and vitality decreases in these moments. We carry that state into the next moment, and the next moment. We start to feel like we're not really living anymore.

It might take time for you to see the cost. It's not always immediate or perceptible in the moment. But it accumulates over time. You don't just stop breathing and tighten up and then forget about it and move on with your life. If you're not resolving the tension in your body, it's creating another open file in your mind. If I make you remember someone or something painful, and then I change the topic, that memory and feeling don't just go away. It's an open browser tab.

We think that non-acceptance is easier than acceptance, but that's only because we've never realized the price we pay with our own life. I'm not telling you to accept or not accept the circumstances of your life; I'm just telling you to do whatever is easier.

I'm a pragmatist at heart. I don't want you to follow some ancient philosophical principle for its own sake; I want you to do whatever is easiest for you in your life. What's easier, acceptance or resistance?

Let's look at the other side now. If you were operating from *acceptance* of this person or situation, what would your life look like? Not the situation, or the other person's life, but *your life*. Let's say you have to commute two hours to work every day from Orange County to Santa Monica. Moving isn't an option because of your kids or because you can't afford it. Every single day, twice a day, you're operating in resistance to your commute. But if you were operating from acceptance, you would stop bitching every day about the traffic. You'd savor the opportunity for alone time, or maybe you'd find a new podcast to get excited about. Or maybe you'd step it up and have the difficult conversation with yourself about whether it's time to look for a new job. Sometimes acceptance means looking at reality in the face and finally making the changes you've been avoiding with all your stories and excuses.

I'm a pragmatist at heart. I don't want you to follow some ancient philosophical principle for its own sake; I want you to do whatever is easiest for you in your life. What's easier, acceptance or resistance? It seems on the face of it that non-acceptance is the easiest thing. We don't want to accept something that's less than perfect; we want to change it! We want to get rid of it, fix it, make it better! Or we just don't want to deal with it at all.

We may think that accepting means being passive, just giving up. But this is not what I'm talking about. Acceptance isn't giving up. It's not resignation, and it's not weakness. A mind in acceptance is about action. It's resistance that's passive. When we resist, the mind may be active, but the body is passive—meaning that your mind is analyzing, efforting, fighting, but you're not actually doing anything about the situation, perhaps because you don't have the energy. Turn this principle around! Become aware. Keep the mind relaxed and accepting and the body dynamic. With the mind in acceptance, life force goes up, the body is at ease, and we can act from a place of greater awareness, with much better chances for success.

Acceptance doesn't mean sitting there and taking the punches; it means ending the internal war against reality that you've been fighting for your entire life. Raise up the white flag, surrender to the "enemy," and accept the life that's in front of you. Now you're ready to get up and kick ass!

The Power of Active Acceptance

There's so much confusion about the word *acceptance*. We don't really understand what it means. Doesn't the word itself just make you feel a bit bored? Does your mind start drifting off as soon as I mention it? Do you decide that it's a good time to zone out? Notice that. It comes from a common misperception about what this word *acceptance* actually means and the power it contains.

Acceptance is one of the oldest words and the most important spoken by the ancient masters in many traditions, including the Greeks. Socrates talks about acceptance. All of the ancient masters agreed: resistance is a sign of weakness, and acceptance is one of man's greatest strengths. When you surrender and accept, you seize the opportunity to rise above the challenges.

We tend to think that acceptance is for pushovers, that it's for the lazy and unmotivated. It's for those spiritual types who sit around and talk about peace and love but don't actually do anything to change the world. Leaders don't accept, they fight, right? Successful people don't accept life as it is; they bend and shape reality to fit their will! That's what we've been taught. It's accurate, but only to the extent that the "fight" is not in the mind. What we don't realize is that the outward "fighting" and creating we do from a place of internal acceptance is *infinitely* more powerful than the uphill battle we're fighting from a place of internal resistance. We can choose to use our time and energy for fighting an impossible battle *against* what is, or we can gather our resources and *respond* to what is. Acceptance is so powerful because it comes from a place of being completely in the present moment, with a quality of honesty, openness, and directness with oneself. This makes us a wide-open channel; it sends life force through the roof. In acceptance, you become endlessly more powerful.

Accepting is not about letting people do whatever they want with no consequences. It's not about standing by and doing nothing in the face of injustice or suffering. What we're talking about is the mind becoming centered so that you can move and act from a clear perspective of "this is how the situation is." When you reach that place, you will have the energy, clarity, and access to your innate intelligence that will help you to make the right decision about what to do next. That voice of *I hate this, I don't like this, It shouldn't be this way* has a lot of emotional charge to it. So much energy is consumed mentally that you don't have enough left to take meaningful action. In acceptance, that voice goes silent. Rather than getting stuck in endless loops of thinking, you simply act as the present moment requires.

It's much more powerful to create change from this place. It reminds me of a mother I worked with who lost her child in a school shooting several years ago. Today her whole will, her life force, is focused on the goal of ending gun violence and making sure no parent has to suffer the way that she suffered. She got active and went to work advocating for new legislation, awareness, support groups, and a broader cultural conversation. She is taking dynamic action toward change. Before she could reach that point, she had to go through her own grieving process and accept that she lost a son. She had to come to terms with the fact that her child is gone. Now, to the degree that she centers herself around the overwhelming magnitude of that loss and becomes motivated by it, she will be able to create change. Otherwise, her actions will be nothing more than emotional uproar and reactivity. I'm not saying the emotion shouldn't be there. I understand and empathize with her pain. It's a loss bigger than anything imaginable. But in order to use the power of that emotion and energy toward something constructive, she has to accept that her son died a violent and unjust death. She cannot become an effective champion for others until she accepts that. In the same situation, another parent lost a child and is still questioning years later if things could somehow have been different. That parent isn't able to fight constructively—only to fight against what is.

When I tell you to accept, I'm not telling you not to fight. Please, fight for what you believe in! The very culture that came up with this notion of acceptance, meditation, yoga, and loving-kindness is a place that also has a legacy of warfare. In the Bhagavad Gita, one of the most important and widely read works of Indian philosophy, the warrior Arjuna is in resistance himself—he is resisting fighting a war against his own kin. The epic poem opens on the battleground where Arjuna will fight his cousins and uncles and family members whom he loves so much. He rides his chariot into battle against his own family to fight for what's right after being guided by his guru into acceptance. This kind of acceptance isn't about peace and love and rainbows and puppies. No. For the sake of being an effective warrior for change, you must first accept there is no other option but to fight.

The Gita was a constant companion and source of strength for Gandhi—the original peaceful fighter—throughout his life. He called the text his "eternal mother." It became not only an inspiration to him but a practical guide to life and service. The central teaching of the Gita, according to Gandhi, was "acting without attachment": doing whatever it is we are called to do without concerning ourselves with the results of our actions. This is just another way of saying "act from acceptance," whether that action is raising the white flag or riding into battle.

In war, a good strategic general is effective because he sees the full picture of what's happening and makes a clear-minded decision in acceptance of *what is*. He risks because he is committed to being "happy"—that is, to a positive outcome—not committed to avoiding "unhappiness," or difficulties. Here's an example from more recent history: In the battle of Dunkirk in World War II, 300,000 Allied troops were backed up against the English Channel and completely surrounded. There was no way out. It would take months for military boats to get to them, and the Germans were a very short distance away. Many in the British government wanted to surrender to Germany in order to save the troops. They were committed to avoiding difficulty, not to making things better. The impulse to surrender might seem like a kind of acceptance, but it's really just resignation based in fear, which is not what we're talking about here. In true acceptance, there is clarity to see the big picture. Churchill had this clarity—he saw and accepted the terrible situation his troops were in, and he assessed the terrible price of surrender. He thought on his feet, with total clarity and deep insight, and realized that if he sent 800 or 900 private boats out to Dunkirk to load up the soldiers, then there was a *chance* that they could get them out safely. Meanwhile, he had to look past the rest of England saying, "You have to surrender; don't let 300,000 of our men get killed." Churchill was moved to action from a place of clear acceptance. This is the state of mind that we're talking about. "The purest, clearest state of mind under pressure" is another way to understand acceptance.

As Churchill wrote in his war memoirs, "United wishes and good will cannot overcome brute facts. . . . Truth is incontrovertible. Panic may resent it. Ignorance may deride it. Malice may distort it. But there it is." In other words? He's saying, "Don't resist the truth; face it instead." From there, a "eureka" moment arises that tells us exactly when and how to pick up the sword and fight. This is the power of life force in action. It's operating from a state of flow, with the energy of life itself at our backs to support and guide our actions.

To help you move from resistance to acceptance in your own life, whatever truth you are facing, here are some simple awareness-boosting exercises to try.

EXERCISES: Breaking Down the Walls of Resistance

1. The most powerful way to move from resistance to acceptance is through some soul searching. The first step is to become aware of what parts of your life are operating with resistance, as well as rejection, denial, avoidance, and the like. Get a journal. Start having an honest conversation with yourself about what you're resisting and what it's costing you. Give yourself a wake-up call. When you become aware of your resistance, it deeply and instantly opens the mind to greater possibilities and transformation.

2. Resistance is usually an indication that your mind has narrowed in its perception. You're stuck in a fixed position. Stop and write down what you're telling yourself about why something happened—for instance, getting passed over for a promotion: *My boss has never liked me.* Then give yourself four other possible reasons why you didn't get promoted. Create four other possibilities and write them down. They don't have to be real or true, and you don't have to believe them. You create these possibilities in order to save your own mind and stop losing energy. Considering other explanations for why things are the way they are can help you to stop pushing your mind into fixed positions and open yourself to freedom from what you're resisting.

3. Try a similar exercise when you feel resistance against something that might happen in the future. On a piece of paper, list four potential outcomes of the situation other than the one you're anticipating and fearing. What else might come of the situation? Imagining a few other possibilities will help you get unstuck from a fixed mental position of anticipating the worst. It's how you can change your intention and make a more clear choice for your next step.

CHAPTER 12

Cutting Craving

If you've ever watched a child throw a temper tantrum, you know exactly what craving looks like. A child in the throes of a kicking and screaming fit wants something so badly—a toy, an ice cream cone, whatever—that it's as if their mind and body have become completely consumed by the object of their desire. Children in the throes of a tantrum look like they've been possessed! They'll yell and scream, "Nooooo!!! I want it now!! Give it to me NOW!!" They will not stop until they get what they want or move on to another toy. The worst tantrums end with the parent throwing in the towel because they've gotten so fed up. Or the child moves on to wanting something else. On occasion, the tantrum ends because the child has gotten tired for the moment . . . but only for the moment. The child will be back, full on, after a short nap to recover the necessary gusto.

As you're reading this, don't fool yourself into thinking you've grown out of this kind of behavior. We grown-ups suffer from the "gimme gimmes" just as much as, if not more than, small children. Adults throw tantrums all the time! The only real difference is that we learn not to do it in public or even to show it in private, so we appear to have better control over our desires. Instead, we wear our "crazy" on the inside, throwing tantrums in the privacy of our own minds. Our minds can easily become possessed by desire in the pursuit of what we want. In this state, we burn through our life force more quickly than a flame burning through an oiled rope. Now, I know your mind is telling you right now that going after what you want with single-pointed focus is an act of determination, and there's nothing wrong with that. I agree with you—but only so long as you're not losing your peace of mind (or your sleep) over it. At that point, it's not determination but your inner "crazy."

Close your eyes quickly and think about something you really, really want—something that your happiness, or even just your *okayness*, depends on. It could be a house, a job, an ideal body weight, the fulfillment of a goal or dream, a life partner. If there's nothing you're craving that strongly right now, think back to a time in the past when you wanted something so badly that it hurt. The wanting became more powerful than you. What happened to your mind? It zeroed in on the object of desire, excluding all else. When the mind is in craving, all of our attention and energy is going toward *I want it, I want it, I want it.* What do I want? *THAT.* When do I want it? *RIGHT NOW.* Emotions intensify, racing of thought increases, clarity and coherent judgment are lost. We call desire "blinding" because it renders us unable to see or focus on anything except for the object of our desire. There's a total loss of perspective. Nothing else matters!

This mind-set has a profound effect on your health, relationships, career, happiness—in short, every aspect of your life. If you pay attention to what's going on physically in craving, you may initially notice sensations similar to those of resistance: a tightening in the chest, shortening of the breath, tension in the muscles. It's the body in a state of non-acceptance. You can't accept the fact that you don't have what you want, and your entire body is tightening up in protest. But there's something else going on too. If you keep exploring this inner experience of craving, you'll start to notice a strong sensation of heat rising. Think of it as the heat of desire.

Adults throw tantrums all the time! The only real difference is that we learn not to do it in public or even to show it in private.

Physically, emotionally, mentally, and energetically, what craving does is build heat. When desire is especially strong, we say it's *feverish* because the temperature of the entire system is literally rising. The fluids in the body, all the nerves, arteries, and energy channels, start to boil up. It's what we call a *burnout*. Think about what happens when you heat elastic things, like rubber—or, in this case, arteries and energy channels. They get loose and floppy. Energy starts to leak out. What you're doing is melting down and burning through your own life force. You're leaking out vital energy, and you will quickly lose the stamina, endurance, and resilience you need to go after what you want. You're becoming loose and floppy! I don't think you need me to tell you that this isn't the best state for being dynamic in life.

We've talked about resistance as a slow cancer that dulls and drains us over time. Craving, on the other hand, is a fast burn that spreads like a wildfire through the whole system. Huge amounts of energy are exerted both to fuel the fire and to cool down the system so that it doesn't boil over. Highly ambitious people (myself included!) are at high risk for burnout because, as we've seen, ambition—which is nothing more than a desire to achieve one's goals—easily tips over into craving. The energy of ambition can fuel and motivate us in the short term, but if we don't balance it with rest and release, we end up running out of fuel when we're only halfway through the race. It's fast-burning energy that can power us through a sprint, but it's not ideal for running a marathon.

Life isn't a sprint. Your career, your family, your most important goals are not a sprint. Accomplishing anything meaningful is a marathon, requiring steady, stable energy that lasts over time. It requires stamina and resilience, which are expressions of life force. The ability to endure and persevere comes from stable life force, not from the energy of a kettle boiling over.

On the mind level, craving creates a kind of tunnel vision. It keeps your attention zeroed in on a fixed goal and a fixed way of getting there. The blinders of desire prevent you from seeing any other goal or way of doing things. Craving attaches you not only to the outcome you're seeking but also to the way of getting there. You're so focused on the path you've decided is the right one that you're not open to alternatives. When something gets in your way, the system moves into attack mode. You start to overreact to setbacks because you don't know how to redirect. To achieve success in going after what you want, you have to remain open because sometimes you can get to Rome a different way. But the mind in craving doesn't want to find a different way. It says, *I know what I want, and I know what I need to do to get it. Now get out of my way.*

Letting Go of the Goal

On a quantum level—on the level of what we create and attract in this unlimited field of possibilities called "life"—the energy of craving blocks the flow of life and abundance. Life can't share its riches with you, the way it naturally does, if you insist on holding on so tightly to what you want and ignoring everything else. Have you ever noticed that when you're desperate for something to work out, it usually doesn't? It's a little joke that life plays on us: When we're so fixated on needing something to happen, the thing we want is often withheld from us. But the moment we say, *F*ck it, I don't even care anymore. It can happen or not happen. I just want to relax and enjoy my life*—that's when it comes. It's the woman who finally lets go of her need for a romantic partner and decides to embrace life on her own, and then suddenly bumps into the love of her life at a coffee shop a month later. It's the couple who can't think about anything but starting a family but has been unable to conceive for years. The moment they let go of the goal and decide to just enjoy being a family of two—the moment they say, *It will come if and when the time is right*—the pregnancy test comes back positive.

This is how the so-called law of attraction really works. While your intellect is focused on the object of your desire, the deeper and much more powerful layers of the iceberg are focusing on the lack of it. Your emotions, your memory, your subconscious mind, and your beliefs are all repeating, *It's not here. I can't have it. I'll never have it.* And as we know, the submerged iceberg is much more powerful than the tip. What's happening in the subconscious is what you're creating. A mind-set of lack, even if it's subconscious, materializes more lack. It's that simple. Meanwhile, the universe rewards a state of relaxed neutrality in going after what you want.

There's nothing wrong with having a goal, but in order for the goal to materialize itself, you have to let the mind be free of the goal to a certain extent and come back into the present moment.

I have a dear friend who's created a beautiful life for herself. She's achieved a lot of success doing what she loves, she's getting more new clients than she can handle, and she lives in a gorgeous apartment in Manhattan. She has an active social life with many good friends, and she's close with her family. But her mind is only focused on the one thing she doesn't have: a relationship. She's on every dating app, and for years she's been going on two or three first dates every week without fail. Her desire to find love is so strong that the experience of dating and meeting people has become clouded by her own feverishness. In the process, she is blocking the very outcome that she wants. Her mind is so fixated on the goal of getting married that she doesn't give herself a chance to really see and get to know the people she's meeting. On every first date, she immediately sizes up the man with an eye toward her end goal. It's no mystery to me that she hasn't met someone yet! Now, I'm not saying that she shouldn't go after what she wants, but it's clear how her craving is standing in the way of her goal. With her mind stuck in her desire, her authenticity and spontaneity are gone. If she could let go of the goal and trust that what she desires will come to her in time, she would be more open and at ease when meeting someone new. She'd be less guarded and better able to have fun and get to know people in a natural way. And if there were something she could do differently to increase her chances of success, she'd have the clarity and mental agility to figure out how to change her approach.

What craving does, again, is narrow your vision. You lose track of the big picture. You stop trusting, and you start trying to control everything. You stop flowing and you start forcing. Life is lost, energy is wasted, outcomes are worse. There's nothing wrong with having a goal, but in order for the goal to materialize itself, you have to let the mind be free of the goal to a certain extent and come back into the present moment. You have to get out of the future that you desire and act from what's here right now. You need to mobilize all your juice, your energy, your intellect, all your skills and talents, to move toward the goal with grace and flexibility.

When Is Desire Too Much?

Desire can be a healthy, positive force in life. But how do you know if you've shifted from healthy desire to destructive craving? It's when the goal becomes bigger than you. That's what happened to my friend: finding a husband became bigger than her happiness, her self-worth, her ability to enjoy life, and her peace of mind. In her mind, it was more important than her ability to appreciate the life she'd worked so hard to create.

You can also identify when healthy ambition tips over into craving by how well you sleep or don't sleep, the quality of your interactions with the people in your life, and how you're attending to self-care and other important aspects of your life. You know it, you feel it, you just choose to ignore the signals. The number one signal that your desire has reached red-alert status is this feverish quality we've been talking about. Think about what a fever is. It's defined as "an abnormally high body temperature, usually accompanied by shivering, headache, and in severe instances, delirium." There you have it. Craving is a state of delirium in which you start to lose track of everything—yourself, your health, your friends, your family, your well-being—because you've been so overtaken by desire. Your mind fills with hot emotions: annoyance, frustration, anger, agitation, hostility. You won't rest until you get what you want.

The Voice of "Not Enough"

Craving keeps us running on the hedonic treadmill, forever unsatisfied with what we have. It's the voice of "not enough." The cruel irony is that, even when we do manage to get what we want, when we finally achieve our dreams, we're not happy. It's still not enough. Look at someone like Steve Jobs. He was a man with so much ambition, and he used it to create some of the most groundbreaking innovations of recent decades. But his ambition also got the best of him. According to the people who were closest to him, Jobs was not a very happy person. People who knew him said that he never stopped to appreciate his achievements and give himself a pat on the back. After a product launch, he was back at work at 6 A.M. the next morning as if nothing had happened. Nothing he accomplished was ever enough: not building Apple into a multi-billion-dollar company, not the Mac, not the iPhone. Through the sheer force of his ambition, he burned himself out, he burned out the people around him, and ultimately, his system broke down and he became ill. Is this what success looks like to you? Please note, I am not suggesting that anyone stop working hard or innovating. I am saying the mind doesn't need to be burned down as you create and innovate.

When you're able to hold your life in a bigger perspective, desire is a positive force that pushes you forward. You want your business to succeed, but it doesn't swell up so much in your mind that it pushes out all the other needs, desires, and demands of your life. With healthy desire, you can still see the big picture clearly. You can think with clarity; you can play around with different ways of achieving your goal without getting stuck in any one thing. If it doesn't work out, you create a new goal and dream a new dream. You find the other roads to Rome.

When desire is healthy, you remain vibrant regardless of whether or not you achieve the goal. You have more stamina and ease in going after your goal because your happiness and self-worth aren't resting on it. You'd like your business to succeed, but if it doesn't, life will go on. Sri Sri often says that if your self-worth, if *who you are*, becomes smaller than the goal, then you know you're stuck in feverishness. If you make the success of your start-up the outsized goal, then the value of your business becomes greater than your own value. The goal has become bigger than you! You've lost your own power and self-worth. You've forgotten that you are so much bigger than anything you accomplish. If the goal were actually bigger than you, then you wouldn't be able to accomplish it, right? When you maintain this awareness of your own power, your own majesty, and your own potential as you go about pursuing your goals, an enormous amount of vitality and attraction opens up and becomes available to you.

With healthy desire, you can still see the big picture clearly. You can play around with different ways of achieving your goal. If it doesn't work out, you create a new goal and dream a new dream. You find the other roads to Rome.

Putting Out the Fire

The first key to overcoming craving, as we've said, is simple awareness: *Am I stuck in craving right now? Have my happiness and self-worth become dependent on this goal? Has the goal become bigger than me?* When you can see that you're operating from craving, something immediately shifts. When you can say to yourself, "I'm really craving this thing right now," a cool breeze of air comes in and turns down the heat on the entire system. Tension releases, breath cools down, thoughts flow toward stillness, and mind-set widens. The boiling in your system reduces to a simmer, and eventually that simmer calms down to room temperature. As soon as you see and recognize craving for what it is, it stops being craving. The goal stops being bigger than you.

And as within, so without. Making this internal shift will quickly lead to external shifts in your life. When you let go of the need for things to work out a certain way, that's when things seem to come to you without effort or forcing. The universe supports that wide-open, relaxed state of mind. It's a natural state of magnetism. As soon as you're able to say, *It's okay, it's all going to work out,* things almost immediately begin moving. You may have to say it more than once. You may have to repeat it many times. It all depends on the size of the craving. But you will find that people start getting back to you. Obstacles start clearing. If in the midst of the craving you can take a little time-out to say, *Everything will work out in the end, I'm just going to chill out,* you widen your mind-set. You feel lighter and more energetic instantly! In that moment you tap into a vast reservoir of energy.

This energy is not mechanical, as I've said; it's a nurturing, supportive life force. It's what gives us life in the biggest sense: the quality of connection, joy, love, vibrancy, creativity. It's the feminine force that wants to serve and uplift us. When we relax and trust that life is taking care of us as a mother takes care of her children, then that force can serve us. That energy surges into the system. All the arteries, energy channels, muscles, organs, and cells relax, and life can flow through once again. Connecting to this energy is as simple as holding the awareness of *Whether I get what I want or not, it's all going to work out.* I know it's not easy to get there and it can be even harder to stay there. But it is very possible, and we must begin somewhere.

Energy Is the Key

Awareness is the first step. The next secret is to maintain a positive mind-set of acceptance by keeping our energy levels high. This is when we return to the basic wisdom at the heart of Vedanta: *Increase your energy.* You already know that when your energy is high, your mind-set and perspective naturally widen. Just as children are most likely to throw tantrums when they've missed a nap, we are more likely to get stuck in craving when we're tired. When you start losing yourself in the pursuit of a goal, come back to your breath. Your meditation. Take a walk in nature. Get a solid night of sleep. If you haven't taken a vacation in a year, get away for a long weekend. The goal will quickly come back into perspective. Consider a weekend retreat at the Art of Living Center in the beautiful Blue Ridge mountains. It's mind-blowing.

When a friend came to me at a point of total desperation from a heartbreak, I taught her some breathing and meditation to practice every day. After a couple of days of practice, when her energy got back up to a healthy level, her perspective changed. She started feeling lighter, more confident, and more relaxed, and it literally changed her face. She looked different. The tension in her jaw relaxed and she pursued her goals with more centeredness.

Notice how these two mind-sets that we've been discussing reinforce each other: craving to resistance and vice versa. When you're craving something, you can also see it as being in resistance to the reality that's in front of you right now. And when you're operating from resistance, you're chasing after something "better" than what's in front of you right now. Either way, the result is the same: life and energy are lost, and even if we do manage to achieve our goal, we're not any happier for it. But with high life force and an accepting mind, we rise above the push-pull of resistance and craving.

EXERCISES: Cutting Your Cravings

1. This first exercise is about awareness. Grab a pen and a journal, and take five minutes to write about the role that craving has played in your life. Look back at your life and ask yourself if craving has ever taken over your mind. If the answer is yes, examine the situation and how it made you feel. Look to see the cost and the reward of it. Were you happy after you achieved what you were craving? How long did the happiness last?

2. In the single-minded pursuit of our goals, we can easily lose our lightness, joy, and spontaneity. When you find yourself stuck in craving, consciously work some play time into your day or week. Play without competition or agenda, whatever that looks like to you, whether it's playing with your kids or your dog, taking a dance class, or going to see a comedy. Whatever it is, give yourself real time to enjoy the simple, innocent pleasures of life without ambition or agenda.

3. Get out of your own head by doing something for someone else. Volunteer at an animal shelter or spend time talking to people at an elderly home. It's not about giving money but giving your time, your heart, and your Self to a larger purpose than the goal you're stuck in.

4. Another way to get out of your head and open up your perspective is to simply perform menial tasks. Stop obsessing and do something with your hands! Clean out your desk, garage, or closet; wash your car by hand; plant some herbs in your garden—anything that keeps you focused on a simple physical activity.

Part V

THE BIG

MIND

CHAPTER 13

Undivided Mind

All the mental obstacles we've been discussing boil down to one single problem: we refuse to accept life *as it is*. We are unable to accept that there can be no happiness without sadness, no pleasure without pain, no success without failure, no life without death. This fundamental non-acceptance is the single most difficult challenge we face as human beings. It's what causes us to live, do, and achieve smaller than who we really are. It's what takes our unlimited potential and squeezes it into a tiny box of finite possibilities.

The nature of life is duality, and if we look around, we will see that the polarities that divide us internally are woven into the very fabric of the world we live in. If you observe the basic structure of life, from the macro to the micro, it is held together by pairs of opposites. At a micro level, an atom is made up of a proton and an electron. It needs both a positive and a negative charge in order to exist. At the macro level, the world we see is also made up of pairs of opposites: hot and cold, up and down, day and night, light and dark, happy and sad, masculine and feminine, even resistance and craving. Everything in life has its opposite, and that opposition is required to give it value. Think about it: Can there be hot without cold? The answer is yes, there can, but you wouldn't know it as hot. You need to know the experience of cold to be able to recognize the hot. In between these two poles, of course, there's a spectrum of relative values, like boiling, warm, lukewarm, and cool, but it can ultimately be broken down in terms of these polarities.

A further observation reveals that these pairs of opposites actually coexist in harmony. Imagine the movie *Star Wars* without Darth Vader. The entire balance of the movie and its plot is gone. As strange as it seems, the evil of Darth Vader is required in order to give recognition to the goodness and courage of Luke Skywalker. Although they appear to be in opposition, the two in the context of the movie complement each other. Only with the presence of both characters in the movie can the movie as a whole itself exist. The same is true for the Harry Potter movies. Lord Voldemort is as necessary as Harry Potter, and vice versa. One without the other is not just an incomplete movie; it's a completely different and much less exciting movie. Without the complement of each other, the characters lose their value.

All the mental obstacles we've been discussing boil down to one single problem: we refuse to accept life as it is.

In life, there is health and disease, war and peace, love and hate, dark and light, pleasure and pain. We will never reach a point of having only one side of the coin and eliminating the other. It's simply not possible. Without conflict or disturbance, you will have no way of recognizing peace or harmony. When conflict disappears, so does the whole notion of peace! Why? Because the mind perceives through the lens of relativity. It cannot recognize anything without its contrasting element. If you had never seen a mountain in your life—not even a photo—and you had no idea what a mountain was, then you would have no awareness of the fact that you live on flat land. You wouldn't be able to recognize it, just as a fish can't recognize water because it's never been out of water. For the fish, there is no *not-water*. But the moment you see the mountain for the first time, the contrast allows you to recognize and experience the flatlands.

This is the way the universe is set up. It's all just a movement of energy up or down, from one pole to the other. This is what we call *polarity*. It's the dual nature of life. Life cannot and will never be one-sided. Nature isn't lopsided! It exists in perfect balance and harmony.

As you've learned, in the Vedic tradition, the two unseen fundamental forces of the universe are *Shiva* and *Shakti*. *Shiva* is the masculine force of pure consciousness, while *Shakti* represents the feminine force, the energy that animates consciousness and brings it to life. The mythical marriage of *Shiva* and *Shakti* represents the coming together of opposite forces that make up the whole of life. It's the Yin and the Yang, the stillness and the activity, the seen and the unseen. Vedanta says that the universe exists in this dance of Shiva and Shakti, as a never-ending cycle of birth and death and rebirth.

Defying Gravity

Here's a question to ask yourself: How often in life do you find yourself fighting against *this basic reality*? How often do you find yourself wishing that there were no conflict, or unhappiness, or poverty, or disease, or war—that there were only peace or happiness, or health, or compassion? Or that you could put a stop to some troubling situation or condition in your life? How often do you tell yourself that everything would be great if only you could get rid of this one negative thing?

What we refuse to accept, what we struggle to even understand, is that life is made up of these pairs of opposites. The root cause of all our troubles is this: *Non-acceptance of life's duality.* To the degree that we cannot accept this fundamental reality, we get pulled into craving and resistance, and to that degree we create a huge drain on our own life force and potentiality.

Most people spend a lifetime of effort and energy running after one side of the equation and fighting against the other. You want to experience only the positive side of life and never the negative. Isn't it true? We are in an endless pursuit of happiness. Unfortunately, this pursuit is a losing game unless we can embrace unhappiness as part of the rules of the game. After all, it's the fight against the opposition that makes the game more fun.

The fact that life is made up of opposites is not the problem. The problem is that the mind has declared war against duality. Mind is on a mission to have only what it wants and none of what it doesn't want. We strive to avoid negativity and seek only positive experiences. Somehow, we've actually convinced ourselves that it's possible! Reality check: this is not possible and it never will be.

I don't mean to belabor the point here, but you have to understand that opposing forces are innate to our existence. Polarity is the substratum of the visible world, the foundation of everything we see, touch, hear, and feel through our senses. It's the two opposing forces together that make up the whole. Life as we know it cannot exist without this duality. Imperfection is part of perfection. And in this indelible truth lies our freedom to do, be, and thrive.

These opposing forces are something we're born into. What is *not* innate, what's learned as we grow up, is the struggle either for or against each of these forces. It's a learned, conditioned response. From the time we're very young, we're taught to chase after what we see as the positive side of life and to run away from the negative. It starts out in childhood with wanting ice cream and not wanting vegetables. As we grow older, it turns into wanting success and happiness and not wanting failure and hardship.

The earth is round, water is liquid, and gravity keeps us tethered to the earth. These are facts! I would love to be able to fly, but unfortunately, there is this thing called gravity that keeps me on the ground. This may be a reality I don't like, but it would be crazy for me to walk around and say, *I hate gravity. Why is there gravity? I wish there were no gravity. I'm going to try to get rid of it.* What an enormous waste of energy and brainpower!

When we try to run away from life's hardships and struggles, it's like picking a fight with gravity. If anybody, anywhere, tells you, "Do this and you'll be happy all the time," the best thing to do is plug your ears and walk away. I don't care what kind of guru or life coach or positive psychologist this person claims to be—they're selling you snake oil. Happiness doesn't come from chasing positivity and running away from negativity. That's self-avoidance. The other option is choosing not to fight with gravity. It's a limitless acceptance of the whole of life.

Again, the acceptance I'm talking about is not passive. It's the most centered and dynamic acceptance from which we create change while keeping our peace of mind. We do what we can to change the world and create all that we want without the desperateness and self-judgment. We live like we once did as children, totally free and in the moment.

So how do we step out from and stand above the push and pull of the opposites?

Option 1: Awareness and Acceptance

Deeply realize the futility of your thoughts and your struggle against life's duality. This allows you to bring your awareness back to the nature of reality in life AS. IT. IS.

I would love to be able to fly, but unfortunately, there is this thing called gravity that keeps me on the ground. It would be crazy for me to walk around and say, I hate gravity. Why is there gravity? I'm going to try to get rid of it.

Once we accept reality, we are home free—not that it's easy to accept. After all, resisting reality is a habit we have been carrying around with us all of our lives. For myself, I find that acceptance comes when I really examine the cost of fighting a losing battle. This brings an immediate transformation in how I think, feel, and act. My mind and my entire nervous system relax. Again, don't start thinking that acceptance makes you passive. Just the opposite: you conserve your energy and resources, and you already know the huge benefits of that. You bring greater clarity into any situation. You return to your center. You shift your emotions from negative to positive. Your outlook gets wider.

When you accept the opposites, you move into the wholeness of life. You *transcend* the pairs of opposites. When you feel sad and you accept it as a part of life, judgment about the emotion itself stops. That allows the emotion to pass through without leaving a lasting scar on the nervous system. Emotions in and of themselves are neither good nor bad. They are just movement of energy. It's the judgment about the emotion that creates the downward spiral of past and future. Any emotion is healthy as long as it comes and goes. When we accept the cycle of sadness or any other emotion, it completes faster, leaving us free from its impact. Suddenly you're a happier person. You are able to weather the ups and downs. Even if it's just the surface of the intellect saying, "This sadness is part of life," you have made a start, because, in that very moment, you've pressed the pause button on the flow of that emotion. Now you have the opportunity to use one or more of the tools we've been discussing throughout the book: change your breath, move your body, use one of the meditation exercises, or take inventory of cost and reward. These "intellectual" pauses may feel slow when you're just starting. That's fine. The results are incremental. The good news is they build at an exponential rate. Each time you pause the emotion, you are breaking the cycle of conditioned response at the base of the iceberg. You are rewiring your subconscious.

Remember that this force of dynamic energy and intelligence is nurturing and life supporting. Please, use it! It wants to support your intention and attention. By moving, pausing to step out of the negativity, and dipping into the positivity, you become the driver of your own creation.

Option 2: Look More Deeply at What Brings Happiness and Unhappiness

If that approach seems too difficult to begin with, then try this one: simply start to observe in your daily life how anything that brings happiness one moment can bring unhappiness the next, and vice versa. One scoop of ice cream brings pleasure and the next scoop not so much, while a gallon later, it brings pain. A boyfriend or girlfriend makes you happy when you fall in love and then brings misery when he or she breaks your heart. You're full of joy and excitement when you buy the BMW you've been yearning for, and then you're exploding with anger when you pull out of the driveway two days later and someone smashes into you. Anything that brings pleasure can bring pain, and the opposite is also true. Getting divorced or fired from your job can bring immediate hardship but ultimately pave the way for the greatest happiness you've ever known.

The point is that the pain or pleasure is not inherent in the object. It's in the perception of your mind as it pushes or pulls. The cycle of life is neither good nor bad. It is what it is! If we really understood this, then we wouldn't resist what we consider unpleasant or negative. We'd stop exhausting ourselves running after the positive. We'd remain centered through the ups and downs. This is what it means to be whole.

When you know, when you *really get it*, that life is made up of duality, then you naturally start to see through a wider lens. You know that everything moves in phases, so you stop fighting against the natural rhythms and seasons of your life. Wholeness means we accept that we're going to have ups in life and we're going to have downs. If you embrace the down cycle and walk right into it with your head held high, it will pass much more quickly than if you resist it. When you try to avoid negativity, it doesn't go away. Instead, it gets tucked into the tissues and cells of your body, and it goes on draining your energy.

This is the Vedic understanding of opposite values: The emotion of happiness, on some level, is a phase. It will pass. Sadness, too, will come, and it will go. It's when we try to avoid one part of the cycle and stay in another that we get stuck. This is why people find themselves in their 50s and 60s still saying that the reason why their lives didn't turn out the way they wanted was because of something their mothers did when they were seven years old. When you try to avoid the down cycles, instead of moving through them, you only stretch them out, and this takes even more of your time, your energy, and your life.

A Whole New Mind

This brings us to the very heart of the teachings of Vedanta (and Buddhism, for that matter): unity of mind. It's nonduality (*Advaita*), meaning "nondual" or "the oneness principle." We're talking about an integrated, synthesized mind. If you recall, this is what *yoga* means: "to yoke," "to unify," "to bring together into an undivided whole." A state of yoga is a total integration and synthesis of the mind. The whole purpose of the practices of yoga is to help us achieve transcendence of the pairs of opposites.

In Vedanta, nonduality or oneness is the single biggest key to unlocking our life force. You may have figured out by now that this idea of oneness and integration is actually something we've been discussing for the entire book, although we've been calling it by different names. Another word for a unified mind is *acceptance*, another word for acceptance is *presence*, and another word for presence is *flow*. It's all connected. What we're talking about, again, is a mind in the present moment. This is the Big Mind.

In so many traditions, monks and sages describe the deepest state of meditation as this kind of integration: mind is present, whole, one with the flow of life. It's a blissful, loving state. Think about what happens to your mind when you're falling in love: it coagulates. The division melts away. People who are newly in love experience such an explosion of energy that they feel as if they could do anything. They feel invincible. This is exactly what's happening when an artist "becomes one" with his or her work in a state of intense creative flow, or when the yogi reaches the state of "single-pointed mind." In the present moment, mind, body, spirit, and environment are coming together as one.

You are a whole that is so much greater than the sum of its parts. Out there in the world you experience through your five senses, there's duality and separation, but internally, the essence of who you are is oneness.

The idea of "oneness" might sound pretty esoteric, but it's a psychological principle too. Where Vedanta talks about accessing the wholeness that is our nature, positive psychology talks about self-actualization: overcoming inner conflicts and struggles to fulfill our deepest potential as human beings. Abraham Maslow, the first psychologist to define self-actualization, described it as "an unceasing trend toward unity, integration, or synergy within the person." This is simply a modern retelling of the wisdom of the rishis: *Unify your mind to unlock your potential.*

Both Maslow and Vedanta agree that the more divided the mind is, the more we lose our dynamism and potential. A divided mind is more stuck in the negative past and more caught up in resistance and craving. It causes us to move away from the positivity and power that are at our core. We start living from this limited box of the conditioned mind, which is *not* who we are. It's only the mask we wear. Living from this narrow mind-set means lower life force, reduced vitality, being out of flow, feeling cut off and separate from life. Our energy and potentiality get fragmented and scattered. We feel that we've somehow "lost" ourselves, and it's because we've shifted our center of gravity away from the unity at the center of who we are.

You are a whole that is so much greater than the sum of its parts. Out there in the world you experience through your five senses, there's duality and separation, but internally, the essence of who you are is oneness. To return to that essence, we're introducing a powerful awareness of the dual nature of life as well as a mind-set that allows us to transcend that duality. Whenever we return to that awareness, all layers of the iceberg, each of the seven faculties of the system, come together in harmonized action. This is where our energy, our potentiality, operates at its maximum.

The Power of Commitment

To understand how a divided mind is draining your energy, think about it from the perspective of energy and vibration: If you hold two conflicting thoughts in your mind, what do you think happens? The universe will support both, but only halfway. It will support the positive outcome you want as well as the negative outcome that you anticipate and fear. This is a recipe for lukewarm results. In life, you have to commit 100 percent. You have to go all in! Don't hesitate; don't hold back; just make a choice, follow through, and if necessary, redirect yourself as the moment requires. You have to move forward in one direction and one direction only. If you're running a race, you don't look at the other 12 runners and wonder if you should be doing it more like them. You just run as fast as you can! We create powerful results in life when we are fully committed to what we want to create. This is a single-pointed mind. You're not waffling back and forth; you're committing to what you're doing and centering your mind around that commitment.

When the mind gets stuck in doubt and uncertainty, we drain our energy and potential. *Should I do this? Should I do that? What if it doesn't work out? Is there something else I should be doing instead?* The mind becomes paralyzed by choices. We think that the more options we have, the better off we are, but this isn't true for the mind. Too many choices drain our power. Think about how many choices you have anytime you walk into the grocery store. Choosing between 12 different kinds of toothpaste takes up not only a lot of time but also a lot of brain power—certainly more than the choice is worthy of! This is what psychologists refers to as the "paradox of choice": the more choices a person has, the more stress that person will experience and the less action that person will take.

Anytime you're stuck going back and forth about something, or when you're doing something but you're only in it 50 percent or 80 percent, you create confusion and produce murky outcomes. In the Yoga Sutras, Patanjali says that if you want to get rid of obstacles, *eka tattva abhyasa*: "have your awareness on one thing." Make your mind single-pointed. *Just do one thing, and don't question the other options or potential problems.* What he's describing is the power of commitment. When you are 100 percent committed to something, resistance and craving fade away because there is acceptance of the whole. When you are dead set on launching your dream business, you're in it come hell or high water. You don't avoid or deny the challenges. You don't look at your competitors and wish you had what they have. No. You embrace all the ups and downs as necessary parts of the larger whole that is your true goal and your vision. Whenever we are completely committed to something in life, we experience wholeness.

Real commitment in the journey of marriage means that you accept the highs and the lows of life together: for better or for worse, in sickness and in health, for richer and for poorer. Perhaps with sex or no sex—yikes! Let's not go that far. But in all seriousness, if you are committed only for better, in health, for richer, it's not a real commitment. You are committed 50 percent, and it's practically guaranteed that your marriage will fail. Everything else in life works the same way. We only achieve our goals and discover what we are truly capable of when we commit to something with our whole being. Children naturally do this: they laugh with their whole being, and they scream and cry with their whole being, then they move on to the next moment with a fresh mind. There is so much power in this way of living. What we don't realize is that there's more power in our wholeness than there is in just our positivity. To be whole, we need to realize the darkness is only the absence of light.

Being Okay with the Not-Okay

As I said earlier, I don't believe in self-improvement. It's an oxymoron. If you look at life through a wider lens, you understand that everything—including you—is created with this dual nature, so there's nothing to fix. There's nothing inside of you that's *not* supposed to be there.

How easily we forget that being a human means being a part of nature. That means that the nature of life—beautiful, wild, creative, and destructive—is mirrored in our own nature. Who we are is made up of opposites. The basic fact to remember, and not to fight against, is that nobody is "perfect" without the imperfection. Enlightenment includes ignorance, even if it's just a drop in the ocean.

Still, the intellect likes to categorize, label, and judge everything. So we divide our emotions, experiences and personal qualities into the categories of right and wrong, good and bad, positive and negative. *This part of me is okay, and that part is not okay.* Then you're on a mission to fix that not-okayness. You forget that there's an entire ocean of possibilities within yourself, and you just get stuck on the one or two little drops that you don't like. When you can take a wider perspective and accept yourself as a whole, the tendencies in you that you'd like to reduce automatically quiet down and disperse. They become just another drop in the ocean. This is the opposite of what happens when you keep fixating on the "negative" trait, which makes it become a thicker and thicker groove in the mind. Instead of being a little crack in the wall, it becomes a deep canyon.

What would it be like to relate to yourself from a mind-set of wholeness? Try this for a moment by bringing to mind some of the qualities you don't like about yourself. What do you consider your biggest flaws? What are the parts of yourself you're always fighting against or trying to fix or overcome? Is it your self-doubt? Your lack of motivation? Your loneliness and isolation? Your bad temper? Your relationship struggles? Your traumatic childhood? Bring two or three of these qualities to mind and sit with them for a few minutes. Contemplate these aspects of yourself with curiosity and list the value of each quality in your life. It might take some time, but if you reflect for long enough, you will eventually see that the things that are "not okay" in you have actually served you in some bigger or more powerful way than the immediate negative impact you tend to focus on. That "thing" has helped to make you stronger, more resilient, more agile, or more compassionate. Maybe it's taught you something about yourself or about life. It led to mistakes and failures that helped you change your approach. If you can see this larger positive value in your not-okayness, you will stop fighting against your "lesser" qualities. And when you stop denying and fighting against them, it's so much easier to learn from them and create an even greater positive outcome. If you can see your not-okayness as something that has the ability to serve you and to hurt you in equal measure, then you can go about the work of self-change and self-improvement from a place of acceptance and compassion rather than one of judgment, rejection, and resistance.

Through the lens of wholeness, we can see that many of the things we consider weaknesses are actually some of our greatest strengths. Perhaps you've always felt like you don't belong; you've carried a feeling that you just don't fit in. How might that have served you? Not fitting in with the herd has a way of challenging people to stand tall in their individuality and work harder to create a life and community that fits their uniqueness. The world would be deprived of some of the greatest works of art, literature, and music if all of these outsider creative geniuses just tried to be like everyone else! The pain of being an outsider can hurt you, or it can become fuel for creation and self-expression. Those brilliant creative minds had to learn to embrace who they are and find a sense of belonging within themselves. So we can understand the not-okayness of "not belonging" as something that has served a positive purpose in helping you carve out your own unique corner of the universe instead of trying to fit into someone else's. Ultimately, from the field of oneness and nonduality, there is only belongingness. We are all the same at our core. We are part of one family: the human family.

---

*Who cares if there's this one annoying thing
about yourself that you can't seem to get rid of?
It's okay! The sky will not fall down. Can you
be kind to this part of yourself and try to
peacefully coexist with it?*

Widening the lens through which you see yourself brings true compassion. Buddhism so often talks about "loving-kindness," or *metta*, practice. For most people who start exploring this practice, it's very easy to direct love and compassion toward others. The Buddha says, however, that the place to start is with love and kindness toward oneself. This is a much more difficult task for most people. It's easy to love your good traits, but it's not so easy to love the pain, struggle, and not-okayness. Here, again, the answer is to widen the lens. Remember that you are a part of nature as much as the trees and the clouds and the birds and bees. You didn't pop into the world as a screwup while everything else is in perfect order! You are a part of all that is, a critical piece of the whole. You have to trust that in nature, even when the big trees block the light for the small trees and make it harder for them to grow, there is some symbiosis happening in the ecosystem. A lion in the forest kills one animal, eats once, and sleeps for practically six months afterward. That preserves life in the forest. For the lion to try to be anything other than what it naturally is would throw off that fragile balance.

The not-okayness is there in you because of some okayness; because of the negative, the positive side of you is ultimately enhanced. Your struggles are bringing something greater to your life. If you have this attitude, then you will see the positive qualities within yourself flourish. You'll move through the negativity more smoothly and learn its lessons more quickly. You will naturally evolve into a greater whole, supported and propelled by your more difficult qualities. But that can't happen when you're either pretending that your difficult qualities aren't there or constantly telling yourself, *It's not okay, it's not okay, it's not okay.*

I often have students who come to me and say, "There's this terrible thing about myself, and I just can't seem to change it. I've spent 10 years meditating and going to therapy, and nothing helps." My answer is always, "So what?" So what if you have this bad habit or negative quality! Who cares if there's this one annoying thing about yourself that you can't seem to get rid of? It's okay! The sky will not fall down. The heavens will not rain fire on you. Can you be kind to this part of yourself and try to peacefully coexist with it? Instead of trying to change it, can you agree to live with it? It's fine! I bet it's not nearly as bad as you think. Look at the whole universe, and get some perspective. If this one thing is your biggest issue, you're doing pretty well. In fact, you're great. Just let it be there, and don't worry about it so much. Know that this thing is a part of your karma: it brings a lesson or teaching. There is always a larger plan at play, even if you can't see it.

The mind has to expand in order to be supported, nurtured, and uplifted by the dual force of life that we call *Shiva* and *Shakti*. Getting stuck in loops of "God, I can't fix this thing about myself" or "I can never get this right" or "I wish I could just be like that" is the tightest, most shrunken mind-set there is. Know with all your heart that it's the crack that allows the light to come through. Stop holding on so tightly to your struggles! Embrace the beautiful, messy whole that is your Self in its fullness.

CHAPTER 14

It's All Connected

We've come full circle to the question that started this whole journey: *Who am I?* The question that led me, step by step, from my cultural identity to the very center of my being. *Who am I at my core? What makes me "me" in my essence? What do I have in common with all that exists, with this world I live in, if anything at all?* These are not questions for empty philosophizing. I use them to this day as a practical means of accessing the greater potentiality of who I can be. It's a way of exploring my larger cosmology and its impact on my daily life.

If we want to understand who we are, it's important to go back to the beginning—back to when we were created. Both science and Vedanta have deeply investigated the question of how the universe was created and how it evolves. Although they use different language, they've arrived at strikingly similar hypotheses. For now, we'll use the vocabulary of science that's more familiar to us. What science tells us is that 13.7 billion years ago, the fiery eruption of the big bang exploded the universe as we know it into being. Time and space came into existence, and then, when the universe was only about three minutes old, the explosion cooled enough for the very first particles of life and matter to begin to form.

These particles were known as *atoms,* the basic building blocks of all matter and all life. In Greek, *atom* means "indivisible," because it was once believed that atoms were the smallest units of matter in existence. Of course, now we know that if you break down an atom, you'll find that it's made up of even smaller units. An atom is created with three different types of subatomic particles that are pulled together by a magnetic attraction. The very center of the atom, the nucleus, is made up of a mix of *protons* (particles with a positive electrical charge) and *neutrons* (particles with no electrical charge). Circling around the periphery of the atom, bound to the nucleus by an electromagnetic pull, are negatively charged particles called *electrons*. What we know is that in every atom, the core has a positive charge, and the negative charge circles around the perimeter.

Life continued to evolve from these basic particles toward greater complexity. Atoms formed groups called molecules, and from molecules came single-celled organisms, and then multi-celled organisms. From there, bacteria and plant and animal life developed. Animals continued to evolve in intelligence into creatures such as dolphins and primates, and then eventually into humans.

Both science and spiritual traditions have observed that life is always evolving. Growth and change is the nature of all of life. Within human beings, that evolution continues. We find individuals who are in some aspects more evolved, aware, and conscious, like a Nikola Tesla or an Albert Einstein, a Gandhi or a Mother Teresa, a Nelson Mandela, the Dalai Lama or Sri Sri. We could say that these souls operate far beyond the human norm. But just look at how far humanity has come from the Stone Age to the digital age. We are evolving to become the sage, the master, the rishi, the enlightened Buddha, the self-actualized being. We don't need to worry about becoming enlightened right at this moment, but we are interested in tapping into the core of who we are to become more alive, more dynamic, more powerful beings, to be the most highly evolved version of ourselves.

Who am I at my core? What makes me "me" in my essence? What do I have in common with all that exists, with this world I live in, if anything at all? These are not questions for empty philosophizing.

Why did we look back all the way to our creation? Because no matter how complex and highly conscious human beings become, we can still trace our evolution all the way back to those first atoms. Those tiny atoms and you were created from the same source energy. Indeed, what you call *you* is just a collection of an unimaginably large number of atoms full of energy. One hundred trillion of those atoms have to come together to form a single cell of your body, and there are over *37 trillion* cells in the human body—you do the math!

The Center of You

Why this even matters is because you, like the whole of any complex structure, are a reflection of your individual parts. You're what we call a *macrocosm*, which is a scientific theory that can be traced all the way back to the ancient Greeks and ancient India. It means that, on some level, the structure of you as a whole is the same as the structure of your smallest building blocks. So really get this: An atom is made of energy. You are made of trillions and trillions of atoms. That means that you are energy. The Greeks and the Indians said that it also works the opposite way: the micro is a reflection of the macro, meaning the structure of the subatomic world mirrors the structure of a human being, which mirrors the structure of the entire cosmos.

You can learn a lot about who you are as a whole by looking at what you're made up of on the smallest level. What you call "me" shares the same basic structure as the atoms that come together to form the cells that make up your tissues and organs that make up the whole of your human body, mind, intellect, memory, and spirit. What that means—as we've been saying this whole time—is that who you are at your core, just like the proton of the atom, is a positive energetic charge. It's a force of attraction rather than repulsion. It's a kind of magnetism that helps us to create, attract, and manifest what we want in life.

Let's take it a little deeper. The energy that created the big bang, according to Vedanta, was already present in an active state in a kind of bubble. This active state created the pressure in the bubble, and it exploded. The big bang didn't create the energy—it always was. After the explosion, something within that energy created matter and life, from subatomic particles to bacteria to you and me. The question is, *What was it within that energy that allowed for this creation to happen?* How did this whole thing happen? Where did the energy in the bubble come from in the first place? Where did the first sign of life come from?

I don't have the answer, and neither do the scientists. However, for thousands of years, mystics all over the world have said that this energy that exploded to create all things was not a cold, mechanical, random force. They've described it as a dynamic, pulsating field, full of intelligence and the power of life itself. In addition, the rishis say the quality of this force field is creative, nurturing, transformative, and always life-supporting. It is a substance called love . . . not the emotion of love but the principle of love itself.

That energy is what created the atoms that make up all of who you are. You are not just made up of these physical units of atoms. Your atoms, and you, are made of this field of energy and intelligence. We can call it "source power." This power is a field of all possibilities. Everything in the cosmos has come from it. It is a field of love and life in full dynamism, expressing itself and its intelligence as YOU, through YOU. This energy created everything from itself; therefore, all that is created has the same potentiality from which it was created. This energy is the creator, creation, and creativity itself. You are made up of this same substance and the same potentiality and power. You are the source of this beautiful, glorious energy. Within you lies the source of creativity and the ability to create. Dare I say it loud and clear? You are a creator, or at least a *co-creator*, of your own life.

As we've discussed, this source power is clearly evident in a baby. Children are full of energy and dynamism, throbbing with joy, love, and excitement from every pore of their being. The child is made up more of energy and love than he or she is made up of matter. They have an endless amount of energy and innate awareness. It's the child's nature; it's your nature. You are born with it. It never ever leaves you. The events of life cover it, like clouds in front of the sun. For some people, the events are so dense, so traumatic, that the clouds are more like a hurricane. It can take some time for the sun to burn through it all. But burn through it always does.

Going back to the energetic makeup of an atom, remember that positivity is your center. It is your essence, your nature, your core, your nucleus. And you already know how huge the energy of an atom can be—just think of the atomic bomb. That's the power at your core. The electrons that circle around the nucleus are the *periphery* of who you are. That negative charge is part of the whole, but it's not the center. When we keep our attention focused on the negativity, it grows. Because we have the potential to create whatever we put our attention and energy on, we create more negativity. When our awareness is on the negative, our center of gravity migrates away from the core of our being and scatters out into the periphery—into thoughts and emotions of the past and future, conditioned thinking and limited mind-sets, resistance and craving. This is what we experience throughout the system as stress. When we fix our attention on the negative charge, we are creating more of that negativity as a result. There is no need to judge the negativity. Instead, we can simply hold an awareness that no matter how stuck we feel, that thing that's holding us back is *not our core essence*.

No matter how strong it feels, that negative charge is never more powerful than the positive charge. That's not the way atoms work! If you weigh the mass of an electron, you'll find that it's *significantly* smaller than a proton. In fact, a proton is *1,837 times* heavier than an electron—that's the difference between the weight of a penny and a bowling ball! In the same way, your positivity is exponentially stronger and more powerful than your negative charge. What does that mean for your life? It means that you are exponentially more powerful when you create and design your life from the center of your being as opposed to its periphery.

The whole journey we have been taking throughout this book is about peeling back the layers of our periphery in order to return to our center. We have seen how operating in the periphery, from the conditioned mind, drains our energy and created a state of stress in the system, which generates even more negative thoughts and emotions, pushing us even further away from our core. But no matter how long we've spent away from the center of ourselves, we can always begin the journey home to our true nature. That journey is the path of self-mastery and self-actualization. Whether using the practices of the Vedic tradition or any other, what you're doing is removing the masks of the conditioned mind, like peeling back the layers of an onion, until what's left is the core. The incredible secret that the ancients knew is that when we connect to and enhance our life force, the onion skin peels off on its own.

> *You are exponentially more powerful when you create and design your life from the center of your being. The whole journey we have been taking throughout this book is about peeling back the layers of our periphery in order to return to our center.*

Our innate life force is what guides and fuels us throughout the journey. In their scientific observation of the inner world, the rishis started with the outermost layers of their being, following the river of life force inward all the way to their very core. When they reached that core, what they found was this ocean of consciousness, unimaginably deep and powerful. But it wasn't something different from the river. This life force and consciousness were two sides of the same coin: the feminine and the masculine, *Shakti* and *Shiva*, the seen and the unseen side of life. Both are made up of water, particles of hydrogen and oxygen, the river in motion merging into the ocean. They observed that this consciousness, which was also described as pure awareness or intelligence, isn't just some empty, impersonal force. It had the quality of *satchitananda*: unchanging, lively, blissful awareness.

The Particle and the Wave

Now let's look back to the structure of the atom, and this time, we're going to go a little deeper. As our scientific understanding of the world has evolved, we've learned that any atom, any particle, isn't just a particle. It's also a wave. Physicists have proved this with the famous "observer effect." What that means is that when a particle is being observed—when the attention and awareness of the observer is on it—then the particle behaves as a particle, meaning that it occupies space and has a mass to it. But as soon as the observer looks away, the particle collapses into a wave, meaning that it behaves more like pure energy—without mass and without occupying one specific place in space. A wave exists in unmanifested form, as pure potentiality in a field of possibilities.

The rishis also called this field of possibilities the "unified field," or consciousness. They understood it as the very substratum of all that there is to life. It's a field of all-knowingness that contains all information, everything that has ever been and everything that could and will ever be. What the rishis call the "unified field" is what a scientist might refer to as *singularity*, or the elusive "theory of everything": the single force underlying all reality that science has long been searching for. I would love for science to discover the basis of this unified field, but to me, that's like the fish trying to recognize the ocean. The fish has to step out of the ocean to recognize itself *and* the ocean, which is impossible. The fish and the ocean exist as one. Remove the ocean, and all you have is a dead fish. But the ocean can go on existing with or without the fish. It will just be more still, with fewer movements and ripples.

The unified field is what connects all of life into a single, indivisible whole. When religions and wisdom traditions talk about "oneness"—which Vedanta calls *Advaita*, or nonduality— they're making reference to some version of this unified field of consciousness. If a particle is a drop of water, the wave is the ever-changing individual or event in the field called "ocean." Who you are is the particle and the wave, a drop of the ocean and the ocean itself. You are both an individual, separate being and an inextricable part of the whole of life.

It's easy for us to forget our interdependence and interconnectedness. In the search for individuality, and in our conditioned, separatist point of view, we forget how everything in our lives is connected with someone or something else. The simple reality is that we are dependent on each other for our survival. The simple act of eating involves an entire ecosystem. Someone has to plant the seed, someone has to tend to it, grow it, pick it, transport it, sell it, buy it, cook it, eat it, and digest it with the help of an internal team of gut microorganisms. When we first came into the world, we operated predominantly from the unified field of consciousness. We hadn't yet identified ourselves with this body, this upbringing, this personality, this limited identity. We didn't look out of our eyes with separateness, isolation, fear, and limitation; instead, we looked out of our eyes with these loving and expansive qualities of the field of consciousness, *satchitananda*. That's what we're getting back to: who we are at our core, the way we were when we were born.

You know by now that when we speak of energy, we are also speaking about consciousness. They are one and the same. When you enhance your energy, you are also expanding your consciousness. We focus on energy because it's something that we can more easily access and control through physical processes, and it changes our consciousness as a result. As our energy increases, we get closer to that unified field. As energy shifts from its more gross, outer form to its more subtle manifestations, we move toward the qualities and power of consciousness. The gross aspect of energy is expressed physically as mass, and in the mind, it's expressed as a sense of separation, negative emotions, non-acceptance, thoughts of the past and future—in short, all that keeps us small. The subtle expression of this energy is a sense of belongingness, love, expansion, positivity, clarity, acceptance, presence, resilience, collaboration. It's what the rishis call the "Big Mind."

As energy increases and consciousness expands, we become more and more powerful. We access more and more of the positive charge within the center of the atom.

From the Stone Age to the Quantum Age

As human consciousness evolves, our understanding of the world is shifting from a particle-only perspective to a broader view that can embrace the duality of the particle and the wave.

For most of human history, a particle-based understanding of reality has dominated in the West. We had to start with the *seen* world before we could make our way to the *unseen*. Science as we know it began when humans first started observing the material world around us, labeling and organizing the objects we saw, and making explanations and predictions. It makes sense: with eyes open, we are looking outside. So why not make sense of what we see? In the East, however, science and spirituality worked side by side. One asked, *What is this?* and the other asked, *What am I?* Where science left off, spirituality began. In the West, the two were kept strictly separate. Scientists separated the head from the heart.

Western science started out with the grossest material elements of life and moved on to the more subtle. With Isaac Newton, particle physics was born. Newton said that "everything is matter"—all there is to life is what we can see, hear, touch, and feel. At that time, everything was understood in terms of matter, separation, division, and multiplicity. The universe was seen as a machine-like entity that operated mechanically according to a set of physical laws.

This Newtonian understanding of life was limited, but it paved the way for science to evolve in a more subtle direction. After Newton comes Einstein, who looks beyond matter to energy and light, time and space. Then physicists such as Planck and Bohr pick up from where Einstein left off and begin observing the quantum level of reality. We move into this idea of wave function, the unified field, and the observer effect. This is where things get interesting. The observer effect proves that the awareness of the observer shapes the observable reality, at least on the subatomic level. Scientists begin to see that when our intention and attention are on something, in a very real way, we are creating that thing. Our consciousness is fundamentally shaping the reality we experience.

Who I am is still a mystery to me, but what I do know is that there is so much more to who we are than what we see with our eyes.

We've moved all the way from Newton to emerging theories of consciousness that mirror what the mystics have been speaking about for thousands of years in India based on their study of the inner world of the mind. Just as humanity has evolved in our understanding of the material world, internally, we are also evolving from an atomized, Newtonian perspective of who we are to something much deeper—an underlying, unifying reality beneath the separate parts of our identity.

I have personally and directly experienced this shift from the particle to the quantum. When I was younger, like so many people, I saw myself as my body, my roles and identities, my thoughts and emotions. My identity was only what I could see, hear, touch, and feel. But once my awareness began to expand into these more subtle aspects of life, there was no going back to my old ways of seeing the world. My own experience of life became my evidence and my guide. I saw how I was connected to everything and everyone else. There was a part of me that was somehow beyond my physical body, my roles and identities, and even my personality, even if I couldn't possibly really understand what it was.

Who I am is still a mystery to me, but what I do know is that there is so much more to who we are than what we see with our eyes. To think that the trillions of cells coordinating their activity in perfect harmony to create the miracle of the physical system that is keeping you alive—orchestrating at every moment your breath, your heartbeat, your neural firings—is a random accident of nature? That's just limited, Newtonian thinking. There is an energy and an intelligence that is moving every breath in and out. Think about it: You need energy in order to inhale, don't you? So what came first, the breath or the energy? For the breath to enter, the lungs first have to expand—it's not the other way around, with the breath entering and the lungs expanding. The movement of the lungs comes first. What made the lungs expand? What is that movement? It's energy, *and* it's intelligence. There is a knowingness in that energy that propels the lungs to expand, breath to come in, and the heart to beat. Your heart is always beating inside of your chest, but what is making the heart beat? The beat itself is life force. You need energy for the heart to contract and then release.

A quantum perspective refocuses your attention from separate, atomized parts of your identity to the greater, unified whole that is your true self and the even greater whole that you are a part of. You know that this foundational force upon which everything is built—including you—is this thing that is a field of consciousness and energy, all-knowingness and pure creative power. What if, just hypothetically speaking, you could see yourself as being a part of this larger force? What if you could see past the particle to the wave underneath? Everything would change! Instead of separation, you'd see connection. Instead of fixed positions, you'd see potential and possibilities.

The Drop and the Ocean

As consciousness evolves—or to say it another way, as energy increases—we become more and more powerful in co-creating with life. At your periphery, where it's all about survival and competition, you can only create within that limited sphere of thinking. But the closer you get to the core, joy and generosity start to increase. Gratitude comes in. Clarity arises. We're moving toward higher expressions of consciousness, which require more energy also. One of the biggest shifts as we move toward the core of our being is that we start to see and embrace the connectivity of life.

I love the words of Leonardo da Vinci, who spent his life bringing together art and science: "Develop your senses—especially learn how to see. Realize that everything connects to everything else." *Learning to see* is exactly what we're doing here. When we change the way we see, we change everything in our lives.

The ancients knew very well that every part of life was connected to the whole in a perfect design. They tell us that there is a purpose and a plan in all things that's larger than we can possibly know. The plants, animals, mountains, and oceans, the stars, the cosmos exist in perfect order. If there were the subtlest of chaos, everything would implode. Trees, flowers, and vegetation grow in the climate that nurtures the fastest growth. The same is true of you and me. Why is it that we as humans remove ourselves from the greater cosmic plan? We do it because we have this added freedom of choice, but that doesn't mean we're outside the design. If we can see the larger design, if we can understand how we're all connected, then we find what it is we're really looking for: to be a part of something greater.

There's no doubt that there's a force of intelligence that's driving everything, the genetics of genetics. We need to be able to look around with wonder at the miracle of life that is occurring all around us. We need to widen our mind-set to take in the bigger picture. Then we can see that there is such an innate intelligence in the plant kingdom, in things like how photosynthesis works, how bees pollinate plants. There is a synchronicity, a coherence, and a harmony with everything in nature, without man interfering on a destructive level—and even that interference will ultimately be rebalanced as a part of life's natural drive to evolve and cohere.

Learning to see is exactly what we're doing here. When we change the way we see, we change everything in our lives.

When you widen your perspective, you cannot help but wake up to the reality that everything is connected. Remember that exercise where you looked at something in front of you, but you were looking *beyond* it at the same time? This is much the same. When you open your awareness to the deeper, unseen reality of life, you start to see beyond the individual particles to the wave underneath. Not only people but all of nature is woven together in an intricate web of interconnection. Zen masters and yogis have been saying this for centuries, and finally scientists are also acknowledging the reality of life's interconnectivity. In a famous experiment, Dutch physicists sent two protons to the opposite sides of a space. They found that when they did something to one proton, it also affected the other proton.[1] In the exact moment, and not a nanosecond later. There was no distance of travel in the impact, not even how long it would take for something to travel at the speed of light. Whether you call this "nonlocality" like the physicists or "interconnectivity" like the sages, we are talking about the existence of a unified field that connects all of life into an indivisible whole. That's why the impact to both protons happens in the exact same moment. This is what gives rise to the empathy that allows us to feel someone else's pain as if it were our own.

That connectivity of life is always there, but we can't see it when our identity is rooted in separateness. When our identity is built on an atomized view of life, we narrow our sense of who we are to our gender, race, religion, and job. But if you really look, even after you describe yourself with all of these roles, you'll see that there is a feeling there is something more. We don't really feel complete in who we think we are because what's missing is our consciousness, this deepest core of ourselves, which is a bigger identity than anything else we could possibly think of.

A child naturally operates from an expanded sense of self, but in adulthood, the mind shrinks to my job, my family, my past, my possessions, my ideas—again, it's the separation, multiplicity, and fixed positions of the Newtonian outlook. Come on! It's time to get past what has already been proven to be an incomplete theory of reality. Welcome to the 21st century—embrace a quantum view of life, and expand your sense of who you are.

Connecting with the Big Mind

The moment you recognize that there is something deeper within yourself beyond all the roles and stories, you tap into the consciousness at your core, into the power of the Big Mind. As a result, energy explodes. You feel invincible! You realize that all these limiting things that you use to identify yourself are changing phenomena. *Prana* increases as you become able to stand on the foundation of a "solid" identity rather than the quicksand of changing roles. Every identity in life is changing, but consciousness is unchanging. That evergreen quality is the *sat* in *satchitananda*. It's what looks out of your eyes that is playing all of those roles but somehow untouched by them. Remember that opposites give each other value, so the only way that you can know change is through the reference point of that which is unchanging and eternal. If you could just recognize that there's something in you that's untouched by all the struggles, the trauma, the bullshit, you would unlock a vast reservoir of energy.

To come back to that larger identity, what you need to do from time to time is look at yourself in the mirror—again, this is the practice we've discussed of looking *at* while also looking *beyond.* Gaze past what you're wearing, your facial features, your hair and skin, directly into your own eyes. Shift your vision to see your eyes one by one. You will want to avert your gaze at first. But if you stick with the exercise, you'll see that you move back and forth to each eye with intentionality. At some point, you may start to realize that you are something behind your eyes, something looking through. There arises the question, *Who am I?* Don't be in a hurry as you contemplate this question. Take your time. Can you see that there is something beyond the way you look, the things you've experienced in your life, and the events that have come and gone? There is something deeper within yourself, something unchanging—something we call the Self.

There is a powerful way to connect to the part of ourselves that is nonchanging even as the body goes through its cycles of birth, growth, decline, and death. You can get a feel for it by taking yourself through a quick mental exercise here. (For the full experience of this meditation, go to RajshreePatel.com and consider taking my online course.) Take yourself on a journey in your imagination, going back to when you were a child of four. Imagine yourself at four years old as clearly and vividly as you can. Then imagine yourself as an 8-year-old, then a 12-year-old, then a 16-year-old, and so on. Eventually you will come to your current age and bring to mind who you are right now. Then you'll move beyond the present and imagine yourself in another few years, then another 10 years, and so on until you reach your deathbed. This exercise can be very powerful. If you really put your energy and focus into it, you will have an experience of this core essence, this positive charge, that we've been talking about all along.

Your awkward, self-conscious 14-year-old self may appear like a different person from your confident, successful 30-year-old self, but isn't there some essence that connects the two? And don't you see that essence when you imagine your 85-year-old self sitting out on the porch in a rocking chair watching the world go by? Events have come and gone—partnerships, heartbreaks, failures, successes, joys, losses. Can you see that the events have shaped you in some way, but perhaps you are something beyond that? There is something evergreen, some essence of you, that has remained untouched through all these ups and downs.

Everything is connected. When you connect to a deeper sense of your own self, then naturally you connect more to the world around you. And in the end, the thing we really want is to be a part of the whole. The moment you have the awareness of connecting to everything in life as one unit, energy awakens within your core. When you can embrace both the multiplicity of life and its oneness, you embrace wholeness, which wakes up the pulse of consciousness and pure energy even more. You feel internally more powerful, more confident, more at ease. You can look at your life and say, *It is how it is right now, but anything can change.*

Turning your focus to the wave function of life shifts at a cellular level the way that things are moving into the mind. You're introducing cracks into the iceberg so that the ocean can flow through. You're transcending the iceberg and moving into the ocean itself. You find that, through your own thoughts and actions, you have the power to move the ocean. There is a ripple effect to all of our thoughts, speech, and actions. It's like the butterfly effect: the flapping of a butterfly's wings in the Amazon can lead to a storm on another continent several weeks later. A tiny change in a vast, complex system can trigger huge effects in other parts of the system. Who you are is so much more powerful than a butterfly—just think how much you can change with your own thought, perception, and action.

As You See, So You Create

Whether you're aware of it or not, you are constantly flapping your wings like the butterfly, impacting and creating not only your life but the life around you. With not only your actions but your thoughts, you are creating and impacting your reality. Your world is created out of your perception.

*I encourage you to ask yourself this:
What is it that you will create in this field
of unlimited possibilities called "life"?*

The rishis said that everything you see, touch, and feel is an illusion because it is all in your mind. They said this long before science had proved that on some level it was true, that there was an unseen reality underlying our seen reality. We now know that this material world is not the total of reality; it's only the very surface. If you can see below the surface, there's so much more that you can create. Think about how an ordinary person looks at jewelry compared to how a goldsmith does. When you look in your jewelry box, you might see a bracelet, a ring, a necklace, and earrings. They're all separate things, on the one hand, but at the same time, they're also all made up of this same underlying substance that is gold. There's value in the ring or the necklace on its own, but the goldsmith has this extra advantage of being able to see the jewelry not only as the single possibility of a ring but also as pure gold with a wide range of possibilities. Our perspective, however, is more limited. We've been trained throughout life to use our intellect to label, judge, and compartmentalize things, to limit our perception to what we can see and touch, so that we can no longer see the gold. There's nothing wrong with seeing the ring, but it's an incomplete picture of reality. When we can perceive more than we see, we can create with more than just what we see.

Everything is perception. That's the only truth we know. Everything we experience in life is a result of our perception. The world as we experience it is relative: we have to compare everything to something else to know what it is. Hard and soft, hot and cold are relative. Because you believe in what you see, to the degree that you believe it, it exists for you in that way. Where your attention goes is what you create in your life. So what if your perception were different? What if you could see the bracelet not only as a bracelet but also as gold? Then you could configure the potentiality of the bracelet to act as the bracelet or to act as pure gold. As gold, you could turn it into a necklace, or earrings, or any other thing. You could make it into a doorknob if that's what you wanted!

If you see the world through the lens of "I can't," then you won't. If you see yourself as "small and limited," then you are. If you see yourself as superior, you will put others down and focus all your energy on competing and winning. If you see yourself as inferior, then you will always be a victim. Our perspective is our choice. We believe, so we create. If you believe you can't, then you won't, and the reasons why you can't or don't are irrelevant. Trying to shift each individual belief is hard work, so why not just shift the center of your identity to the all-encompassing belief of who you are at your core? If you see yourself as boundless, limitless power, intelligence, and potentiality, uplifted by the unconditional support of life at your back, then you can recognize the world as your creative playground. You can use your creative power to shape yourself into any potentiality that you want. This journey is about looking around and slowly recognizing: *Everything I see, touch, and feel is just a partial truth.* It's only one side of the coin. There is more to me, more to what I see, more to what I touch and feel than I am aware of. When you operate from the most powerful belief about yourself, everything in the universe gets behind you to support you.

Self-mastery is about learning to use this power of perception wisely to co-create with life. When our intention is clear and our awareness is uplifted, molecular structures reorganize themselves to give us what we want. That's when spontaneous healing happens. That's when you manifest things. That's when life comes to you rather than you having to run after it. That's when miracles happen. A miracle is nothing more than a powerful intention coupled with an uplifted state of awareness.

As a final moment of self-reflection, I encourage you to ask yourself this: What is it that you will create in this field of unlimited possibilities called "life"?

Last Word

The true journey of vital force is the movement from *I* to *we*. It's the power of our unity as human beings. It is the power of the wholeness, peace, and potential within each of us, the loving vibrational force of who we, who you, truly are. The more love, peace, fullness you enjoy, the more you move toward the center of your identity, the more this energy ripples out to everyone. The starting point is you.

Becoming liberated from the belief that you are an incomplete, separate being that needs fixing allows you to realize how powerful and magnificent you really are. You connect more not only to yourself but to the whole of humanity. Armed with this awareness and tools for living from your true nature, you will effortlessly treat others as your own. Love, peace, gratitude, and the sense that you are an extraordinary and necessary part of the whole—in time these become natural.

The journey of self-knowledge can be both exhilarating and humbling. With or without our consent, it is the one journey we're all in together. In each of us exists a longing for something more, no matter how much fame, fortune, or power we achieve. The external world will never fulfill that longing. In the end, this longing is what's meant to inspire the search of your inner greatness.

What we seek is within. The love, the beloved, and the lover are all within. The creator, creativity, and creation are within. The achievement, the achiever, and the power to achieve are also all within. The perfection of life exists within you, as you. Do not sleep through it. Awaken. Open your eyes and call upon it. See that all you seek can be effortlessly yours as it already exists.

I want to encourage you to pursue your dreams as if anything is possible. As if all that you seek is effortlessly within your reach. Your mind, heart, and hands need to be open and willing to let go of the "stale peanuts" that you hold on to for dear life.

As our world expands in technology, it is shrinking in core human values. Our frantic culture with its pressures and anxiety to achieve is taking us away from the one thing that can save us and the world: our trust in ourselves.

This deep knowing gives you access to your own power and potential during times of joy and times of challenges. It will emanate from within you to the world. You become the tipping point of not only your own life but life on this planet. The starting place, again, is always you.

Know in your heart that change is always possible. To bring it back to the language of science for a moment, research shows that we can change our brains and the expression of our genes by changing our actions, our lifestyle, our thoughts, and our emotions. It's called neuroplasticity: the brain has this phenomenal ability to reorganize itself throughout life by forming new neural connections. What Vedanta teaches is that the biggest impact is created in your brain and perception by looking inward. You have to decide to let go of the past. You have to decide to let go of what may happen in the future. Let go of the ideas and beliefs that give you survival but not living. Let go of the habituated mind-sets of resistance and craving. Anytime you let go, you are agreeing to crack open the tough head. You are melting the iceberg. You are traveling along that river of life energy back to the ocean of consciousness.

This is my wish for you: That you live in a life that is uplifted and nourished by the loving force of life itself that wants nothing more than to serve and support you.

A simple way to do this is by showing up in the moment the way it is, rather than the way you wish it were. Be willing to be as fluid and allowing as water, to flow and change course as life leads the way for you. Be willing to be powerful and gentle at the same time.

The brain cannot change the brain. The mind cannot change the mind. The very thing that gave you life is what can change and enhance life on all levels. Connect to the source of life as the center of your identity, and you will naturally emulate the qualities of the source. Don't make this some big, far-off goal. Start somewhere. Start here and now. When there is an opportunity to love or to separate yourself, embrace love. Where there is an opportunity to be a giver or a taker, be a giver, even though it may feel unnatural and painful as you stretch out of your conditioned comfort zone. In this tiny moment, in the smallest choice to act from your core, cracks in the iceberg will begin to appear. It is through these cracks that light comes in. In time, you will break off and drop large chunks of iceberg into the ocean. You will start to see yourself not as the solid piece of ice but as water, as the hydrogen and the oxygen, the protons and the photons. You will discover the power of the ocean within your own heart. At some unknown moment, you will find yourself living from the field of all possibilities, this energy and intelligence full of more love than you can possibly contain.

This is my wish for you: That you live in a life that is uplifted and nourished by the loving force of life itself that wants nothing more than to serve and support you. That you walk with the knowledge that this force of life is not separate from you; it IS you. That you use your infinite power freely and wisely to create and shape a life of beauty, purpose, connection, and true happiness, not only for yourself but for those who will follow in your footsteps.

More for You to Explore

This book has a lot of tools and practical tips to harness the power of Vital Force. However, words on paper are limiting. Moving toward our essence is one of the most personal and intimate journeys in life. To support and guide you further not only to optimize all the layers of your life but also to deepen your self-discovery, there is nothing like guidance through online programs or in-person sessions.

When you are ready, explore the opportunities below:

- Weekend retreats at the Art of Living Center in the Blue Ridge mountains. Go to ArtofLivingRetreatCenter.org.

- Effortless Vedic meditation (Sahaj Samadhi). Go to ArtofLiving.org

- Project Welcome Home Troops. PTSD programs for veterans and families. Go to PWHT.org.

Don't sell your smile for just anything. It's the best and the most expensive tool you have. Use it!

Endnotes

Chapter 3: Ancient Biohacking

1. Joel Wong and Joshua Brown, "How Gratitude Changes You and Your Brain," *Greater Good*, June 2017; Patrick L. Hill, Mathias Allemand, and Brent W. Roberts, "Examining the Pathways between Gratitude and Self-Rated Physical Health across Adulthood," *Personality and Individual Differences* 54, no. 1 (January 2013), 92–96; Stephen M. Yoshimura and Kassandra Berzins, "Grateful Experiences and Expressions: the Role of Gratitude Expressions in the Link between Gratitude Experiences and Well-Being," *Review of Communication* 17, no. 2 (March 2017), 106–118.

2. Sara B. Algoe and Baldwin M. Way, "Evidence for a Role of the Oxytocin System, Indexed by Genetic Variation in CD38, in the Social Bonding Effects of Expressed Gratitude," *Social Cognitive and Affective Neuroscience* 9, no. 12 (December 2014), 1855–1861.

3. American Psychological Association, "Review of Research Challenges Assumption That Success Makes People Happy," *ScienceDaily*, December 19, 2005.

4. Martin Seligman, *Authentic Happiness* (New York: Free Press, 2002).

5 National Center for Complementary and Integrative Health, "Meditation: In Depth," January 2, 2019.

Chapter 4: A Machine Called Mind

1. Habib Yaribeygi, et al., "The Impact of Stress on Body Function: A Review." *EXCLI Journal* 16 (July 2017), 1057–1072.

2. Arne Dietrich, "Functional Neuroanatomy of Altered States of Consciousness: The Transient Hypofrontality Hypothesis," *Consciousness and Cognition* 12, no. 2 (June 2003), 231–256.

Chapter 5: The Past Is Present

1. Sally S. Dickerson, et al., "Immunological Effects of Induced Shame and Guilt," *Psychosomatic Medicine* 66, no. 1 (January–February 2004), 124–131.

2. Zak Stambor, "How Reliable Is Eyewitness Testimony?" *Monitor on Psychology* 37, no. 4 (April 2006).

3. "30 Years on Death Row: Wrongfully Convicted Man Offers Forgiveness," CBN News, April 2, 2018. https://www1.cbn.com/cbnnews/us/2018/april/30-years-on-death-row-wrongfully-convicted-man-offers-forgiveness.

Chapter 7: The Secret of Life

1. "Relaxation Techniques: Breath Control Helps Quell Errant Stress Response," *Harvard Health*, January 2015. https://www.health.harvard.edu/mind-and-mood/relaxation-techniques-breath-control-helps-quell-errant-stress-response.

2. Sameer A. Zope and Rakesh A Zope, "Sudarshan Kriya Yoga: Breathing for Health," *International Journal of Yoga* 6, no. 1 (January–June 2013), 4–10. DOI: 10.4103/0973-6131.105935.

3. Emma M. Seppälä, et al., "Breathing-Based Meditation Decreases Posttraumatic Stress Disorder Symptoms in U.S. Military Veterans: A Randomized Controlled Longitudinal Study," *Journal of Traumatic Stress* 27, no. 4 (August 2014), 397–405.

4. Emma M. Seppälä, "Yoga, Deep Breathing Used to Address Soldiers' Post-Traumatic Stress," emmaseppala.com, August 16, 2012. https://emmaseppala .com/yoga-deep-breathing-used-to-address-soldiers-post-traumatic-stress-2/.

Chapter 8: Meditation for Busy People

1. Frederick Travis and Jonathan Shear, "Focused Attention, Open Monitoring and Automatic Self-Transcending: Categories to Organize Meditations from Vedic, Buddhist and Chinese Traditions," *Consciousness and Cognition* 19, no. 4 (December 2010), 1110–1118.

2. Frederick Travis and Niyazi Parim, "Default Mode Network Activation and Transcendental Meditation Practice: Focused Attention or Automatic Self-Transcending?" *Brain and Cognition* 111 (February 2017), 86–94.

3. American Association for the Advancement of Science, "New Study Shows Transcendental Meditation Improves Brain Functioning in ADHD Students," *EurekAlert!*, July 26, 2011.

4. American Association for the Advancement of Science, "Research Validates the Defining Hallmark of Transcendental Meditation—Effortlessness," *EurekAlert!*, November 4, 2016.

5. Moby, "Moby on Meditation: 'As a Profoundly Lazy Person, I Appreciate TM.'" *Transcendental Meditation: Latest News & Opinions*, May 19, 2014.

6. Lorenza S. Colzato, Ayca Szapora, and Bernhard Hommel, "Meditate to Create: The Impact of Focused-Attention and Open-Monitoring Training on Convergent and Divergent Thinking," *Frontiers in Psychology*, April 18, 2012.

7. Frederick Travis, 2011. "The Transcendental Meditation Technique and Creativity: A Longitudinal Study of Cornell University Undergraduates," *The Journal of Creative Behavior* 13, no. 3 (September 1979), 169–180.

8. David Lynch, *Catching the Big Fish* (New York: Tarcher-Perigee, 2007).

9. Emily Ionson, et al., "Effects of Sahaj Samadhi Meditation on Heart Rate Variability and Depressive Symptoms in Patients with Late-Life Depression," *The British Journal of Psychiatry* 214, no. 4 (April 2019), 218–224.

Chapter 14: It's All Connected

1. Wenjamin Rosenfeld, et al., "Event-Ready Bell Test Using Entangled Atoms Simultaneously Closing Detection and Locality Loopholes," *Physical Review Letters* 119, no.1 (July 2017).

Index

A

abundance, 164–65
acceptance, 161. *See also under* resistance
acupuncture, 31
adaptogens, 121
addiction, 121
ahimsa (non-resistance), 160–62
akasha, 48
Allen, Woody (analogy), 101–2
ambition, 209, 212–13
ananda (bliss), 142, 154
anger, 82–89, 92, 125–26
antidepressants, 147–48
anxiety, 82, 88–89, 108, 121
aparigraha (non-possessiveness and letting go), 167–68
Arjuna, 203
Art of Living, xx–xxii, 35, 37, 133, 149
Asprey, Dave, 37
asteya (non-stealing and abundance), 164–65
atoms, 237–43
attraction, law of, 211
avoidance. *See* resistance
awareness
   brahmacharya (higher awareness), 165–67
   chit, 142, 154
   of craving, 214–16
   of duality of life, 225–26
   of one thing, 231
   of the present moment, 100
   of resistance, 191–92
   resulting from high mental energy, 10
   vs. thoughts, 185
Ayurveda, 43

B

Beatles, 111
belief
   defined, 26
   limiting beliefs, 34–36, 69
   setting aside disbelief (being open-minded), 25–27
beyond the horizon (exercise), 150
Bhagavad Gita, 90, 138, 184, 203
Big Mind (consciousness), 29, 48, 54–55, 59, 228, 245, 250–52. *See also* consciousness
biohacking, 6, 37, 41–49
blame, 84, 86–87
body
   defined, 55
   energy for, 7–8
   rules of operation, 56–57
body-mind complex, 6–7. *See also* mind
brahmacharya (higher awareness), 165–67
brain. *See also* frontal cortex
brain wave coherence, 141
   energy consumed by, 9
   limbic, 61, 64, 119
   during meditation, 141
   negative bias of, 80
   neuroplasticity of, 256
   transient hypofrontality, 68
breath/breathing, 117–36
   of babies vs. adults, 126
   benefits, 112
   defined, 55
   emotions' connection with, 18, 124–26, 129–30
   energy movement via, 170
   exercises, 133–36

exhaling, 122, 127–128
flutter, 128
gasping for air, 129–30
holding breath, 128–29, 170
inhaling, 122, 127, 247
knowing people through their
    breathing, 127–30
lung capacity, typical use, 124
before meditation, 148–49
and memory, 130–33
mental state impacted by, 112–13
and the nervous system, 118,
    120–21, 132
overview, 117–18
and the power of *prana*, 121–24
relearning, 133–34
and stress, 135–36, 170
Sudarshan Kriya, 121, 133–34
and survival mode, 118–21
British Journal of Psychiatry, 147–48
the Buddha, 110, 158
Buddhism, 110, 139, 157–58, 234
burnout, 63, 209, 213
butterfly effect, 252

C

cancer, 86
children
    babies as happiness, 46–47,
        154–55
    energy of, 14–15, 241
    mind of, 15–16
Chinese medicine, 28–29
chit (awareness), 142, 154
chitta. See memory
Chopra, Deepak, 64
Churchill, Winston, 204
circadian rhythms, 138
collaboration, 165
commitment
    to happiness vs. avoiding unhap-
        piness, 196–98
    power of, 230–31
compassion, 157–58, 234
competition, 164–65
conditioning, 34, 77, 94, 242, 244
connectedness of the universe,
    237–54
    atoms, 237–43
    and the big bang, 237, 240

connecting with the Big Mind,
    250–52
cosmic design, 248–50
    and evolution, 238–39
    and identity, 250–52, 254
    love, principle of, 240
    overview, 237–39
    particle physics to quantum
        physics, 245–47, 250
    particles and waves, 243–45
    perception as creating reality,
        248, 252–54
    the positivity at your center,
        239–42
    and the source power of creation,
        240–41
    unified field, 243–45, 249
consciousness (*Shiva*; masculine
    element). *See also* Big Mind;
    satchitananda
    defined, 55
    evolution of, 245, 248
    and life energy (vital force;
        Shakti), 26–27, 29–30, 41–42,
        242–45
contentment, 171–73
contrary action, practicing, 168–69
craving, 207–17
    awareness of, 214–16
    energy for reducing, 216
    excessive desire, 212–13
    exercises, 217
    heat of, 208–9, 213
    letting go of the goal, 210–12
    as a mind-set, 181–85, 216, 256
    overview, 207–10
    putting out the fire of, 214–15
    tantrums, 207–8
    as the voice of "not enough,"
        213–14
creativity, 12
    and breathing, 128–29
    and flow, 36–37
    in thinking, 145
cultural identity, xiii

D

Dalai Lama, 109–10
depression, 16, 38, 87, 121, 147–48
Devi (divine mother), 39–40

dhyana (meditation), 110–11, 140. *See also* meditation

DNA, 125–26

dreams, 91

duality of life
awareness/acceptance of, 225–26
being okay with the not-okay, 232–35
happiness/unhappiness, sources of, 227–28
non-acceptance of, 223–25
overview, 221–23
and the power of commitment, 230–31
transcending pairs of opposites, 226, 228
and unity of mind (oneness principle), 228–30 (*see also* Big Mind)

Dunkirk, battle of, 204

dwesha (aversion), 181

E

ego, 55

Einstein, Albert, 27, 48, 246

electrical-energy conductors, 189–90

electromagnetic energy (human biofield), 5, 31, 48

emotional intelligence training, 43

emotions
anger, 82–89, 92, 125–26
anxiety, 82, 88–89, 108, 121
and blame, 84, 86–87
breathing's connection with, 124–26, 129–30
and cancer, 86
emotional drain of the past, 81–83
energy used/generated by, 11, 82
fear, 87–89, 197–98
guilt, 84–87
identifying emotional programming, 89–90
negative, 11, 72, 81–82, 125–26
as neither good nor bad, 226
positive, 11, 72, 82
regret, 83–84

engagement, 46

enlightenment, 138, 232

envy, 164–65

exercise, 7–8, 56–57

F

faith in a higher power, 94, 176–78

fear, 87–89, 197–98

feminine energy, 27, 29, 39–40, 215, 223, 242–43

flow
experience of, 24–25
finding, 36–40
intellect during, 68
mind flow, 139, 143–48
resulting from high mental energy, 10

flowing water (exercise), 150

food, 7–8

the Force (from *Star Wars*), 29. *See also* life energy

Freud, Sigmund, 59, 79–80

frontal cortex
activities/chatter of, 62, 97
intellect seated in, 60
rational thinking and strategizing as activating, 107
repetitive thinking in, 70
and resistance, 198
results of temporarily shutting down, 67–68
during sleep, 64

G

Gandhi, Mahatma, 33, 203

gratitude, 45, 82, 93, 173, 248, 255

greatness, inner. *See* superpowers, inner

Greek philosophy, 29, 201

Groundhog Day, 75

guilt, 84–87

gurukula (schooling of mind), xvi

H

hand gazing (exercise), 151

happiness
babies as, 46–47
committing to happiness vs. avoiding unhappiness, 196–98
contentment as, 171–73

as creating success, 45–46
and hard work, xii
pathways to/levels of, 46–47
via positivity, 224–25
sources of happiness/unhappiness, 227–28
harmony
  inner, 168–78
  of opposites, 222
  with others, 160–68
Harry Potter movies, 222
hatred, 161
Hinton, Anthony Ray, 92
human life, layers/faculties of, 54–56
hypnotherapy, 43
hypothalamus, 135

I

IAHV Prison Program, xxi
India
  culture in, xiii–xiv (*see also* Vedic tradition)
  education in, xv–xvi, 48
  yoga and meditation in, 21
individuality, 244
innocence, 169–71
insanity, defined, 76
intellect, 55, 59–60, 62–65, 67–68, 198
intelligence. *See* consciousness
ishvara pranidhana (self-love and faith in a higher power), 176–78
Iyengar, B. K. S., 123

J

Jobs, Steve, 212
journey of self-knowledge, xix–xx, 242, 255

K

Kabat-Zinn, Jon, 106
karma (bondage to the past), 119, 198, 235
kindness, 159, 234
King, Martin Luther, Jr., 33–34
Kozloski, James, 9

L

laying yourself down, xix
leadership, 33–34, 36, 47
Leonardo da Vinci, 248
letting go, 57–58, 167–68, 173, 256
life, effortless power of, xii–xiii
life energy (vital force; *Shakti*), 3–19
  as within and around you, 26–28
  for change, 6
  of children, 14–15
  and consciousness, 26–27, 29–30, 41–42, 242–45
  creative, 12 (*see also* feminine energy)
  defined, xxii
  depleted, 5–6, 13–14, 16, 28
  emotional, 11
  as empowering, xvii–xviii, xxii
  everything as, 48
  feminine, 27, 29, 39–40, 215, 223, 242–43
  as fuel, 4–7
  as heart quality, 190, 193
  high vs. low, 6, 17, 31, 41–42
  hygiene regarding, 169–70
  mental (*see* mind)
  overview, xxv–xxvi
  physical, 7–8
  and quality of life, 5, 10
  sexual, 12–13
  Shakti, defined, 26–27, 39 (see also *prana*)
  spiritual, 12
  success fueled by, 32–34
  tapping, 6, 17–19, 38–39 (*see also* biohacking)
  transformation into matter, 29 (see also *prana*)
  worldwide conceptions of, 28–29
looking through (exercise), 150
Lynch, David, 145

M

Mandela, Nelson, 33, 92
mantras, 138, 143, 146
marriage
  commitment in, 231
  Indian, xiii–xiv, xviii–xix
Maslow, Abraham, 229

meaningfulness, 46
meditation
  vs. mindfulness, 102, 110–11
meditation (*dhyana*), 137–51
  apps for, 139–40
  benefits, 47, 139, 145–48
  brain activity during, 141
  breathing before, 148–49
  defined, 140
  effortless (Sahaj Samadhi), 18, 98,
    112, 138–40, 142, 147–48
  exercises, 149–51
  focused-attention, 140, 145
  in India, 21
  mantras, 138, 143, 146
  mind flow, 139, 143–48
  vs. mindfulness, 47
  mindfulness practice, 98–102
  open monitoring, 140
  overview, 137–40
  self-mastery via, 139
  self-transcending, 140–42,
    145–46 (*see also* Transcenden-
    tal Meditation)
  sleep during, 146–47
  thoughts during, 144–45
  unity of mind in, 228
memory (subconscious; *chitta*)
  and breathing, 130–33
  defined, 55
  energy use, 70
  information stored in, 60–62
  during sleep, 64
  thoughts rooted in, 76–78, 88
  and trauma, 132–33
  mental hygiene, 171
  #MeToo movement, 166
mind, 53–72. *See also* Big Mind;
  brain; consciousness; memory;
  thoughts
  beginner's, 15, 70–71, 171
  vs. body, rules of, 56–59
  of children, 15–16
  conscious, 59–61
  defined, 55
  divided, 229–30
  energy use, xxv, 8–10, 15–16,
    58–59, 62–65, 70–71
  energy-use exercise, 71–73
  vs. the five senses, 123
  as the foundation of your life, 53

intellect, 55, 59–60, 62–65, 67–68
  and letting go, 57–58
mental exhaustion, 8–10
  and old patterns, experiences, and
    beliefs, 69–72
  operation, 59–60, 67
  overview, 53–54
  perception, 55, 59–60
  preconscious, 59–61
  quality of life determined by, 10
  and stress, 65–67
  turning off skepticism, 23
  unconscious, 59
  unity of (oneness principle), 141,
    228–30 (*see also* Big Mind)
mind flow, 139, 143–48
mindfulness, 97–113
  awareness of the present moment,
    100
  being nonjudgmental, 99–100
  defined/characterized, 99–100
  focus, 99, 101–2, 107, 110–11
  how to be more mindful, 103–6
  as keeping us on the surface of the
    mind, 106–8
  as managing the mind, 43
  vs. meditation, 47, 102, 110–11
  mental monitoring, 101, 107–9
  no mind vs. more mind, 110–13
  overview, 97–98
  problems with the practice of,
    99–104, 107–8
  relaxing the mind, 111–12
  rest/calm, 102–3
  resulting from high mental
    energy, 10
  retreats, 108
  stress reduction via, 104–6
  techniques (*see* breath/breathing;
    meditation, effortless; Tran-
    scendental Meditation)
  the zombie effect, 108–10
Mindfulness-Based Stress Reduction,
  106
mind-set
  destructive, 183–84
  repulsion (resistance) vs. attrac-
    tion (craving), 181–85, 216, 256
    (*see also* craving; resistance)
  self-reflection about, 185
  shifts in, 18, 93, 135

mitochondria, 7
Moby, 143
monks, 137

N

negative perceptions, 9
nervous system and breathing, 118, 120–21, 132
neuro-linguistic programming (NLP), 43
neuroscience, 44, 125
Newton, Isaac, 245–46
niyamas (practices), 168–78
  as core essence, 157–59
  ishvara pranidhana (self-love and faith in a higher power), 176–78
  overview, xxvi
  santosha (contentment), 171–73
  saucha (cleanliness, purity, and innocence), 169–71
  svadhyaya (self-examination and self-responsibility), 174–76
  tapas (self-discipline and resilience), 173–74
NLP (neuro-linguistic programming), 43
non-resistance, 160–62
nonviolence, 160–61

O

observer effect, 243, 246
oneness, 141, 228–30, 244

P

panic, 81, 87–88
paradox of choice, 230–31
parasympathetic nervous system, 118, 120, 135–36
the past as present, 75–95
  anger spectrum, 83–89, 92
  emotional drain of, 81–83
  fear spectrum, 87–89, 197–98
  the future as anticipated past, 78–79
  guilt, 84–87
  identifying emotional programming, 89–90

negative thoughts about past and future, 78–81, 83, 92–93
  overview, 75–77
  past and present as not real, 90–94
  the power of the present, 95
  returning to the present, 82, 94–95
  thoughts as rooted in memories, 76–78, 88
  treating the past like a dream, 93–94
Patanjali, 231
  on awareness of one thing, 231
  on contentment, 172
  on faith in a higher power, 176
  on *niyamas* and *yamas*, 157–60, 166
  on purity, 169
  on self-discipline, 173
  on sensory pleasure/sex, 166
  on *svadhyaya*, 176
perception, xix, xxiii, 55, 59–60, 248, 252–54
perfectionists, 86–87
performance enhancement, 43
pineal gland, 135
Planck, Max, 27–29, 246
pleasure, 46, 165–67
pneuma (breath, spirit, or soul), 29. *See also* life energy
polarity. *See* duality of life
positive psychology, 17, 45–46, 229
possessiveness, 167–68
prana (embodied *Shakti*)
  defined, 26, 31
  and identity, 250
  life as made up of, 48
  power of, 30–32, 121–24
  and showers, 170
Psychological Bulletin, 45–46
psychotherapy, 89, 147–48
PTSD, 121, 132–33
purity, 169–71

Q

qi (life-giving energy), 28–29. *See also* life energy
qigong, 31
quantum physics, 29, 245–47, 250

R

raga (attraction), 181
reality
　external (material) vs. internal,
　　xv–xvi
　past and present as not real,
　　90–94
　perception as creating, xix, xxiii,
　　248, 252–54
regret, 83–84
Reiki, 31
relativity theory, general, 48
resilience, 173–75, 209–10
resistance, 187–205
　vs. acceptance, 192–93, 197, 199
　awareness of, 191–92
　committing to happiness vs.
　　avoiding unhappiness, 196–98
　cost of non-acceptance, 198–201
　defined, 189
　and energy conducting, 189–91
　exercises, 205
　letting go, 199
　as a mind-set, 181–82, 184–85,
　　216, 256
　non-resistance as a superpower,
　　160–62
　overview, 187–89
　power of active acceptance, 201–5
　as saying no to life, 193–96
　stress of, 199
　unconscious, 196
responding vs. reacting to situations, 9
rest cycles, 138
rishis
　biohacking by, 41–42
　on breathing, 118, 125
　on getting stuck in the past, 75
　on the layers of human life, 54–56
　on levels of happiness, 46
　on the life force and conscious-
　　ness, 242–43
　vs. neuroscientists, 44
　on raising your vital force, 43
　on reality as illusory, 253
　on returning to the present, 82
　on the unified mind, 141
Robbins, Tony, 33

S

sadhana (spiritual practice), 171
Sahaj Samadhi (effortless meditation;
　dhyana), 18, 98, 112, 138–40, 142,
　147–48
santosha (contentment), 171–73
sat (liveliness), 142, 154, 250
satchitananda (existence, conscious-
　ness, bliss), xxiii–xxiv, xxvi,
　154–55, 243–44, 250
satya (non-changingness), 162–63
saucha (cleanliness, purity, and
　innocence), 169–71
science
　and experiment, 25
　material vs. spiritual, xv–xvi
　physics, 29, 245–47, 250
　and spirituality, 245
secret sauce, 32–34
Self, xxiii–xxiv, xxvi. See also
　satchitananda
self-actualization, 229, 242
self-blame, 84–85, 89
self-discipline, 173–75
self-discovery, xi–xiii, xv
self-doubt, 87, 89
self-examination and self-responsi-
　bility, 174–76
self-help, 18–19
self-improvement, 18–19, 232–33
self-love, 178, 234–35
self-realization, 18–19
self-restraint/self-control, 165–67
Seligman, Martin, 46
sensory pleasures, 165–67
Seppälä, Emma, 133
sexuality, 12–13
Shakti and *Shiva*, 223. *See also* life
　energy
Shankar, Sri Sri Ravi, 187
　Art of Living, xx–xxii, 35, 37, 133,
　　149
　fame/stature of, xxi
　first impressions of, 22–24
　on innocence, 171
　lectures/workshops by, xvi, 22–24
　on preparing for meditation,
　　148–49
　on self-worth vs. goals, 214

stamina and energy of, 109
Shiva, 29, 223
showers, 169–70
Silicon Valley, 37
sleep
    breathing exercises before and
        after, 134–35
    as a cycle of rest, 138
    hours needed, 37–38
    during meditation, 146–47
    recharging via, 7–8
Socrates, 201
sound therapy, 31
spirituality
    defined, 12
    energy used/generated by, 12
    and science, 245
Star Wars, 29, 222
stealing, 164–65
stress
    adapting to, 121
    and breathing, 135–36, 170
    defined, 66
    meditation for, 146–47
    and the mind, 65–67
    mindfulness for, 104–6
    from negativity, 241
    from resistance, 199
symptoms, 135
Sudarshan Kriya, 121, 133–34
superpowers, inner (siddhis), 153–78
    ahimsa (non-resistance), 160–62
    aparigraha (non-possessiveness
        and letting go), 167–68
    asteya (non-stealing and abun-
        dance), 164–65
    brahmacharya (higher awareness),
        165–67
    harmony within, 168–78
    harmony with others, 160–68
    ishvara pranidhana (self-love
        and faith in a higher power),
        176–78
    living your essence, 156–58
    melting the iceberg, 158–59
    overview, 153–56
    santosha (contentment), 171–73
    satya (non-changingness), 162–63
    saucha (cleanliness, purity, and
        innocence), 169–71

svadhyaya (self-examination and
    self-responsibility), 174–76
tapas (self-discipline and resil-
    ience), 173–75
surrender, 177–78
survival mode, 118–21
svadhyaya (self-examination and
    self-responsibility), 174–76
sympathetic nervous system (the
    fight-flight- freeze system; survival
    mode), 118–21, 135

T

tapas (self-discipline and resilience),
    173–75
Tesla, Nikola, 13, 27, 48
theory of everything, 243
therapists, 101–2
thoughts
    vs. awareness, 185
    as electrical impulses, 64
    during meditation, 144–45
    negative vs. positive, 72, 79–80
    number of, 64–65
    the past (smriti) as the root of,
        76–78, 88
    repetitive, 64–66, 68–70
    speech and action connected to,
        159, 163
thriving, defined, 5
TM. See Transcendental Meditation
Tolle, Eckhart, 95
Transcendental Meditation (TM),
    112, 140, 142–43, 145–46, 148–49
transient hypofrontality, 68
Travis, Fred, 141–42
truthfulness, 162–63

U

unified field, 243–45, 249
University of Wisconsin–Madison,
    133
Upanishads, 123

V

Vedas, 29, 42, 45–48, 95, 120–21,
    123, 172

Vedic tradition/Vedanta. *See also*
Art of Living; Bhagavad Gita;
meditation
age of, 43
Buddhism's origins in, 110
on consciousness, 29
effectiveness of, 43–44
on everything as energy, 48
on happiness, pathways to/levels
of, 46–47
on happiness as creating success,
45–46
on innate qualities of humans,
142
on life energy, 26 (*see also* life
energy)
on managing the mind, 42
on memory, 78
on oneness, 228–29, 244
on perception (*manas*) and
intellect (*buddhi*), 59–60
on the positive and the negative,
92
as positive psychology, 17, 45
purpose of, 94
on qualities we're born with,
154–55 (*see also* superpowers,
inner)
on quality of life, 10
for reconnecting to source energy,
44
as a science of the mind, 44
on Self (*satchitananda*), xxiii–xxiv,
xxvi
on *Shakti*/vital force, xxii, 26, 223
(*see also* life energy)
on *Shiva*, 29, 223
on thought as rooted in the past,
76, 88
on yoga, 43–44
violence, 160–61
Vipassana retreats, 157
virtues. *See* superpowers, inner
vital force. *See* life energy
Vivekananda, Swami, 48

W

war, 203–4
Welcome Home Troops, xxi, 133
wellness trends, 43
Wherever You Go, There You Are
(Kabat-Zinn), 106
"Who am I?" (self-discovery), xi–xiii,
xv, 54, 237, 246–47, 251
wholeness, power in, 231–33

Y

yamas (practices), xxvi, 157–60,
162–63, 166, 168
YES! for Schools, xxi
Yin and Yang, 223
yoga
being in a state of, 43–44
breathing, 120–21, 133–34 (*see
also* breath/breathing)
hatha, 44
in India, 21
meaning/goal, 141, 228
Yoga Sutras. *See niyamas*; Patanjali;
yamas
yogic tradition. *See* Vedic tradition/
Vedanta

Z

Zeno, 29

Acknowledgments

This particular time of my life was filled with many ups and even more downs. It was a time when the universe was pushing me to find the power within to lay down and co-create a new reality for myself. This time, and this book, is a testament to the unseen power and intelligence behind everything in my life.

First, my gratitude to that Force that has been by my side, aware of it or not, no matter what I do or don't do.

To say this book is "by Rajshree Patel" is an overstatement. Without the teachings and the unmeasurable love of Sri Sri Ravi Shankar, this book would certainly not exist.

In addition, at the top of the list of gratitude are the countless "Munchkins," "Chotus," and "Chickens" that have contributed to this book, either by their unwavering presence or absence.

I want to specifically thank a few people who were present throughout the birth of this book, including the final push during delivery.

Koesma, for opening your heart and home.

Reshma, for being my eyes and ears.

Sushmita and Pramod, for "adopting" me.

Kanan, for the joy you bring into my life.

Ale, Renata, and my Italian brother, thank you for always saying "yes" and for encouraging me to spread this beautiful wisdom.

Michael Edlestein, for being my "big brother" and keeping me "fed" with all your kindness.

Carolyn Gregoire, for being my hands and holding a "tusk" as you morphed into "Ganesha."

Giles Anderson, for being my voice of reason.

Finally to my family: I love you . . .

Papa, you were my example to live life as a lion, by living it your way. You will be happy to know, you were right. The world isn't black or white. I wish you were around long enough to hear these words in person.

Mama, your enormous sacrifice and resilience are present throughout this book.

Hemant and Sweta, I carry a debt of gratitude for taking care of mom and dad. Your commitment gave me freedom.

Paresh and Chaula, your willingness to risk, to push and care, and always do the best you can, inspires me in ways you may never know.

Kamlesh, I am humbled with awe for who you are, for being a huge loving force of care for each and every member of our family. It gave me the peace of mind to pursue my dreams.

Scottie, I know it hasn't been easy for you to be the "tug-boat," while I disappeared into my cave. Without your resilience, gentle, and silent heart, I could not be where I am today.

About the Author

Rajshree Patel is an international self-awareness coach, teacher, and speaker. She has taught hundreds of thousands of people in more than 35 countries the power of meditation, mindfulness, breath work, and other ancient tools for accessing the innate source of energy, creativity, and fulfillment within.

Born in Uganda and raised between rural India and New York City, Patel was working as a prosecutor for the U.S. Attorney's office and the Los Angeles District Attorney's office when a chance meeting with the renowned spiritual master Sri Sri Ravi Shankar changed her life. She left the practice of criminal law to explore the power of universal laws. She has spent hundreds of hours studying directly with Sri Sri the ancient wisdom of Vedanta. Since then, over the last three decades she has established omre than 600 meditation centers and trained thousands of instructors with the Art of Living, helping expand the self-development and humanitarian organization into a global nonprofit.

Through her unique blend of intuition, humor, and ancient techniques, Patel has guided government leaders, families, Oscar-winning filmmakers, Fortune 500 executives, and individuals from all walks of life in understanding how the mind works, how to let go of stress, and how to be more resilient and fulfilled in their personal and professional lives. She has given talks and led programs at organizations including NBCUniversal, IBM, LinkedIn, Gap, The World Bank, Shell Oil, Morgan Stanley, Harvard University, IIT, the United Nations, UNESCO, and more.

Website: RajshreePatel.com

Hay House Titles of Related Interest

YOU CAN HEAL YOUR LIFE, the movie,
starring Louise Hay & Friends
(available as a 1-DVD program, an expanded 2-DVD set,
and an online streaming video)
Learn more at www.hayhouse.com/louise-movie

THE SHIFT, the movie, starring Dr. Wayne W. Dyer
(available as a 1-DVD program, an expanded 2-DVD set,
and an online streaming video)
Learn more at www.hayhouse.com/the-shift-movie

⌐

*HEAL YOUR DRAINED BRAIN: Naturally Relieve Anxiety,
Combat Insomnia, and Balance Your Brain in Just 14 Days,*
by Dr. Mike Dow

*THE INTERNET TO THE INNER-NET: Five Ways to
Reset Your Connection and Live a Conscious Life,*
by Gopi Kallayil

*YOU HAVE 4 MINUTES TO CHANGE YOUR LIFE:
Simple 4-Minute Meditations for Inspiration, Transformation,
and True Bliss,* by Rebekah Borucki

All of the above are available at your local bookstore,
or may be ordered by contacting Hay House (see next page).

⌐

We hope you enjoyed this Hay House book. If you'd like to receive our online catalog featuring additional information on Hay House books and products, or if you'd like to find out more about the Hay Foundation, please contact:

Hay House, Inc., P.O. Box 5100, Carlsbad, CA 92018-5100
(760) 431-7695 or (800) 654-5126
(760) 431-6948 (fax) or (800) 650-5115 (fax)
www.hayhouse.com® • www.hayfoundation.org

———

Published in Australia by: Hay House Australia Pty. Ltd.,
18/36 Ralph St., Alexandria NSW 2015
Phone: 612-9669-4299 • *Fax:* 612-9669-4144
www.hayhouse.com.au

Published in the United Kingdom by: Hay House UK, Ltd.,
The Sixth Floor, Watson House, 54 Baker Street, London W1U 7BU
Phone: +44 (0)20 3927 7290 • *Fax:* +44 (0)20 3927 7291
www.hayhouse.co.uk

Published in India by: Hay House Publishers India,
Muskaan Complex, Plot No. 3, B-2, Vasant Kunj, New Delhi 110 070
Phone: 91-11-4176-1620 • *Fax:* 91-11-4176-1630
www.hayhouse.co.in

———

Access New Knowledge.
Anytime. Anywhere.

Listen. Learn. Transform.

Listen to the audio version of this book for FREE!

Unlock endless wisdom, fresh perspectives, and life-changing tools from world-renowned authors and teachers—helping you embrace vibrant health in your body, mind, and spirit. With the *Hay House Unlimited* Audio app, you can learn and grow in a way that fits your lifestyle . . . and your daily schedule.

With your membership, you can:

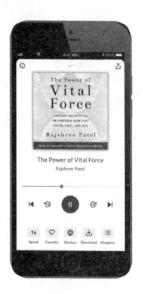

- Develop a healthier mind, body, and spirit through natural remedies, healthy foods, and powerful healing practices.

- Explore thousands of audiobooks, meditations, immersive learning programs, podcasts, and more.

- Access exclusive audios you won't find anywhere else.

- Experience completely unlimited listening. No credits. No limits. No kidding.

Try for FREE!

Visit **hayhouse.com/try-free** to start your free trial and get one step closer to living your best life.

Free e-newsletters
from Hay House, the Ultimate
Resource for Inspiration

Be the first to know about Hay House's free downloads, special offers, giveaways, contests, and more!

 Get exclusive excerpts from our latest releases and videos from *Hay House Present Moments*.

 Our **Digital Products Newsletter** is the perfect way to stay up-to-date on our latest discounted eBooks, featured mobile apps, and Live Online and On Demand events.

 Learn with real benefits! *HayHouseU.com* is your source for the most innovative online courses from the world's leading personal growth experts. Be the first to know about new online courses and to receive exclusive discounts.

 Enjoy uplifting personal stories, how-to articles, and healing advice, along with videos and empowering quotes, within *Heal Your Life*.

Sign Up Now!

Get inspired, educate yourself, get a complimentary gift, and share the wisdom!

Visit www.hayhouse.com/newsletters to sign up today!

HAY HOUSE
Online Video Courses

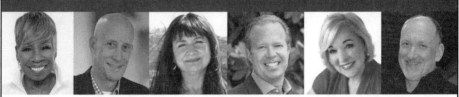

Your journey to a better life starts with figuring out which path is best for you. Hay House Online Courses provide guidance in mental and physical health, personal finance, telling your unique story, and so much more!

LEARN HOW TO:

- choose your words and actions wisely so you can tap into life's magic
- clear the energy in yourself and your environments for improved clarity, peace, and joy
- forgive, visualize, and trust in order to create a life of authenticity and abundance
- break free from the grip of narcissists and other energy vampires in your life
- sculpt your platform and your message so you get noticed by a publisher
- use the creative power of the quantum realm to create health and well-being

To find the guide for your journey, visit www.HayHouseU.com.

HAY HOUSE
online learning